Cynographia britannica: consisting of coloured engravings of the various breeds of dogs existing in Great Britain; drawn from the life, with observations on their properties and uses, by Sydenham Edwards; ...

Sydenham Edwards

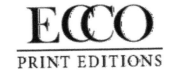

PRINT EDITIONS

Cynographia britannica: consisting of coloured engravings of the various breeds of dogs existing in Great Britain; drawn from the life, with observations on their properties and uses, by Sydenham Edwards; ...

Edwards, Sydenham
ESTCID: T100612
Reproduction from British Library
Published in 6 numbers, the last plates being dated 1805. The text breaks off in the section on the mastiff at the word "Manwood". No more published.
London : printed by C. Whittingham, for the author, Chelsea; and sold by J. White; J. Robson; H. D. Symonds; L.B. Seeley; T. Curtis; and A. and J. Arch, 1800[-05].
8,[72]p.,plates ; 2°

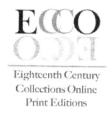

Eighteenth Century
Collections Online
Print Editions

Gale ECCO Print Editions

Relive history with *Eighteenth Century Collections Online*, now available in print for the independent historian and collector. This series includes the most significant English-language and foreign-language works printed in Great Britain during the eighteenth century, and is organized in seven different subject areas including literature and language; medicine, science, and technology; and religion and philosophy. The collection also includes thousands of important works from the Americas.

The eighteenth century has been called "The Age of Enlightenment." It was a period of rapid advance in print culture and publishing, in world exploration, and in the rapid growth of science and technology – all of which had a profound impact on the political and cultural landscape. At the end of the century the American Revolution, French Revolution and Industrial Revolution, perhaps three of the most significant events in modern history, set in motion developments that eventually dominated world political, economic, and social life.

In a groundbreaking effort, Gale initiated a revolution of its own: digitization of epic proportions to preserve these invaluable works in the largest online archive of its kind. Contributions from major world libraries constitute over 175,000 original printed works. Scanned images of the actual pages, rather than transcriptions, recreate the works *as they first appeared.*

Now for the first time, these high-quality digital scans of original works are available via print-on-demand, making them readily accessible to libraries, students, independent scholars, and readers of all ages.

For our initial release we have created seven robust collections to form one the world's most comprehensive catalogs of 18th century works.

Initial Gale ECCO Print Editions collections include:

History and Geography
Rich in titles on English life and social history, this collection spans the world as it was known to eighteenth-century historians and explorers. Titles include a wealth of travel accounts and diaries, histories of nations from throughout the world, and maps and charts of a world that was still being discovered. Students of the War of American Independence will find fascinating accounts from the British side of conflict.

Social Science

Delve into what it was like to live during the eighteenth century by reading the first-hand accounts of everyday people, including city dwellers and farmers, businessmen and bankers, artisans and merchants, artists and their patrons, politicians and their constituents. Original texts make the American, French, and Industrial revolutions vividly contemporary.

Medicine, Science and Technology

Medical theory and practice of the 1700s developed rapidly, as is evidenced by the extensive collection, which includes descriptions of diseases, their conditions, and treatments. Books on science and technology, agriculture, military technology, natural philosophy, even cookbooks, are all contained here.

Literature and Language

Western literary study flows out of eighteenth-century works by Alexander Pope, Daniel Defoe, Henry Fielding, Frances Burney, Denis Diderot, Johann Gottfried Herder, Johann Wolfgang von Goethe, and others. Experience the birth of the modern novel, or compare the development of language using dictionaries and grammar discourses.

Religion and Philosophy

The Age of Enlightenment profoundly enriched religious and philosophical understanding and continues to influence present-day thinking. Works collected here include masterpieces by David Hume, Immanuel Kant, and Jean-Jacques Rousseau, as well as religious sermons and moral debates on the issues of the day, such as the slave trade. The Age of Reason saw conflict between Protestantism and Catholicism transformed into one between faith and logic -- a debate that continues in the twenty-first century.

Law and Reference

This collection reveals the history of English common law and Empire law in a vastly changing world of British expansion. Dominating the legal field is the *Commentaries of the Law of England* by Sir William Blackstone, which first appeared in 1765. Reference works such as almanacs and catalogues continue to educate us by revealing the day-to-day workings of society.

Fine Arts

The eighteenth-century fascination with Greek and Roman antiquity followed the systematic excavation of the ruins at Pompeii and Herculaneum in southern Italy; and after 1750 a neoclassical style dominated all artistic fields. The titles here trace developments in mostly English-language works on painting, sculpture, architecture, music, theater, and other disciplines. Instructional works on musical instruments, catalogs of art objects, comic operas, and more are also included.

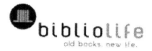

The BiblioLife Network

This project was made possible in part by the BiblioLife Network (BLN), a project aimed at addressing some of the huge challenges facing book preservationists around the world. The BLN includes libraries, library networks, archives, subject matter experts, online communities and library service providers. We believe every book ever published should be available as a high-quality print reproduction; printed on-demand anywhere in the world. This insures the ongoing accessibility of the content and helps generate sustainable revenue for the libraries and organizations that work to preserve these important materials.

The following book is in the "public domain" and represents an authentic reproduction of the text as printed by the original publisher. While we have attempted to accurately maintain the integrity of the original work, there are sometimes problems with the original work or the micro-film from which the books were digitized. This can result in minor errors in reproduction. Possible imperfections include missing and blurred pages, poor pictures, markings and other reproduction issues beyond our control. Because this work is culturally important, we have made it available as part of our commitment to protecting, preserving, and promoting the world's literature.

GUIDE TO FOLD-OUTS MAPS and OVERSIZED IMAGES

The book you are reading was digitized from microfilm captured over the past thirty to forty years. Years after the creation of the original microfilm, the book was converted to digital files and made available in an online database.

In an online database, page images do not need to conform to the size restrictions found in a printed book. When converting these images back into a printed bound book, the page sizes are standardized in ways that maintain the detail of the original. For large images, such as fold-out maps, the original page image is split into two or more pages

Guidelines used to determine how to split the page image follows:

• Some images are split vertically; large images require vertical and horizontal splits.
• For horizontal splits, the content is split left to right.
• For vertical splits, the content is split from top to bottom.
• For both vertical and horizontal splits, the image is processed from top left to bottom right.

COLOURED ENGRAVINGS

OF THE

VARIOUS BREEDS OF DOGS

EXISTING IN GREAT BRITAIN;

DRAWN FROM THE LIFE,

WITH

OBSERVATIONS ON THEIR PROPERTIES AND USES,

BY

SYDENHAM EDWARDS;

AND

COLOURED UNDER HIS IMMEDIATE INSPECTION

Dogs have always been the ready and affectionate servants of man, are excellent companions when human society is wanting, and are the faithful and incorruptible guardians of their master's person and property.—" Dogs are honest creatures, they " never fawn on those they love not, and I'm a friend to Dogs "

LONDON·

PRINTED BY C. WHITTINGHAM, DEAN STREET, FETTER LANE

FOR THE AUTHOR, CHARLES STREET, QUEEN's ELM CHELSEA,

AND SOLD BY J WHITE, FLEET STREET, J ROBSON, NEW BOND-STREET, H D SYMONDS, PATERNOSTER ROW, L B SEELEY, AVE-MARIA-LANE, T CURTIS, ST GEORGE's CRESCENT, AND A AND J ARCH, GRACECHURCH-STREET

1800

INTRODUCTION.

IN the following pages I propose to give a more satisfactory account of the Dogs found in England, with their uses, habits, and appearance, than has hitherto been offered to the public.

The description of each kind is accompanied with a figure delineated from the living animal, which has been attended with great trouble and expence, as it was necessary for the correctness of the work that each portrait should be carefully made from some distinguished individual Dog of each particular breed: and in the execution of the portraits much study and attention has been paid, to represent as strongly as possible the peculiar character and manners of each respective race. Thus far I may venture, perhaps, without incurring the charge of ostentation, to speak of the nature of my labours; the rest is submitted with the greatest deference to the judgment and indulgence of a discerning public.

The descriptive part is occasionally interspersed with some account of the Dogs formerly used in this island, which have been superseded by others more useful, or better suited to the wants or fashion of the times, as may be exemplified in the Blood-hound, which was commonly in use at a period when, as an emblem of war, our restless ancestors pursued the wild boar, wolf, or red deer, on mountainous wastes or wilds covered with forests and thick underwoods, he was employed to trace the wounded game to its concealment, and the midnight thief or blood-stained robber to his secret cave, when our country was cleared, the larger game was destroyed, or only preserved in the parks of our nobles, and the thief or robber found a surer protection in the crowded city than the solitary glen, the services of this animal being no longer useful or necessary, he is lost to us, or suffered to degenerate and sink into obscurity.

In like manner the mechanical arts have superseded the use of the Turnspit, and the introduction of new kinds, with various modes of protecting property, the Mastiff, and other breeds, once frequent, are for similar reasons lost. It would be a matter of great curiosity could their history be pursued to periods more remote; as we might from the Dogs in use deduce the sports and character of times past; but for this I lament the want of satisfactory materials.

The Dog may be considered as, not only the intelligent, courageous, and humble companion of man, he is often a true type of his mind and disposition; the hunter's dog rejoices with him in all the pleasures and fatigues of the chace; the ferocious and hardy disposition of the Bull-dog may commonly be traced on the determined brow of his master; nor does the Dog of the blind beggar look up to the passing stranger but with suppliant eyes.

Always the ready and affectionate servant, an excellent companion when human society is wanting, the faithful and incorruptible guardian of his master's person and property.—— " Dogs are honest creatures, they never fawn on those they " love not, and I'm a friend to Dogs."

England has been long eminent for the superiority of her Dogs and Horses, now preferred in almost every part of the world. Whether this superiority arises from the climate, or from the pains taken in their breeding, education, and mainte- nance, I do not undertake to determine; the Fox-hound and the Bull-dog out of this island are said to lose their proper- ties in a few years; if so, then there must be some local cause of their perfection in this country, and their degeneration in others.

The attachment of our countrymen for ages to the sports of the field has given them health and vigour of body, and a gallant contempt of danger, the uniform effect on those nations that have cultivated them.

Romanis solenne viris opus,
Utile famæ, vitæque, et membris.

HORACE.

The chase was by our sires esteem'd
Healthful, and honourable deem'd.

FRANCIS

Without pursuing these remarks any farther, I will now enter into a short historical dissertation on the Dogs cultivated in this country as far back as any certain account of them can be traced, which is not more distant than the reign of Queen Elizabeth. Of the Dogs existing at this period we have an excellent catalogue from the able pen of the illustrious Dr. Cajus, and according to him there were then known in England sixteen species, or rather varieties of Dogs, for all the different breeds, it is imagined, are merely varieties from one original stock, to which Mr. Pennant and Mr Hunter have added of late years the Wolf, the Fox, the Hyæna, and the Jackall, considering them as offsprings of the same stock. To Dr. Cajus succeed Merret, Ray, Topsell, and Pennant; they have, however, added but little to his invaluable remarks.

The species enumerated by Dr. Cajus are contained in the following table :

NOMINA

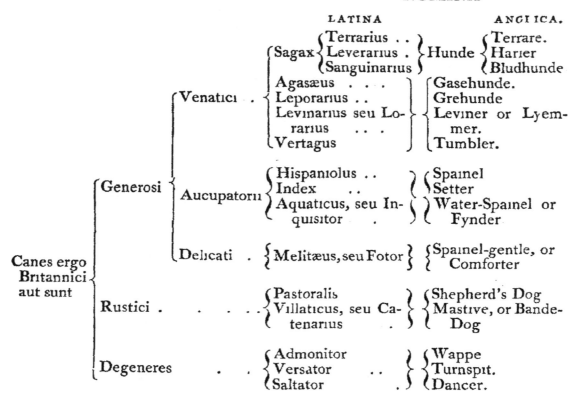

LATINA   ANGLICA.

Canes ergo Britannici aut sunt

Generosi
- Venatici
  - Sagax
    - Terrarius . . — Hunde — Terrare.
    - Leverarius . — Harier
    - Sanguinarius — Bludhunde
  - Agasæus . . . — Gasehunde.
  - Leporarius . . — Grehunde
  - Levinarius seu Lorarius . . — Leviner or Lyemmer.
  - Vertagus — Tumbler.
- Aucupatorii
  - Hispaniolus . . — Spainel
  - Index . . — Setter
  - Aquaticus, seu Inquisitor . — Water-Spainel or Fynder
- Delicati . — Melitæus, seu Fotor — Spainel-gentle, or Comforter

Rustici . . . . .
- Pastoralis — Shepherd's Dog
- Villaticus, seu Catenarius . — Mastive, or Bande-Dog

Degeneres . .
- Admonitor — Wappe
- Versator . . — Turnspit.
- Saltator . — Dancer.

Some of these are wholly extinct, or only a few individuals preserved by the curious.

For the same reasons that some breeds have become extinct, new ones have been formed, and a great number of these changes from fashion and caprice take place in a short period of time; the principal, however, still do, and probably ever will remain.

are termed the permanent, as the mixtures or crosses may be referred to the original races.

The artist also may find these figures useful by exhibiting the outline and character of these animals when the originals are not at hand.

It is hoped the whole will form an useful and entertaining work for the public, and the information given will be collected from the most authentic sources, but chiefly from my own investigation of the different subjects.

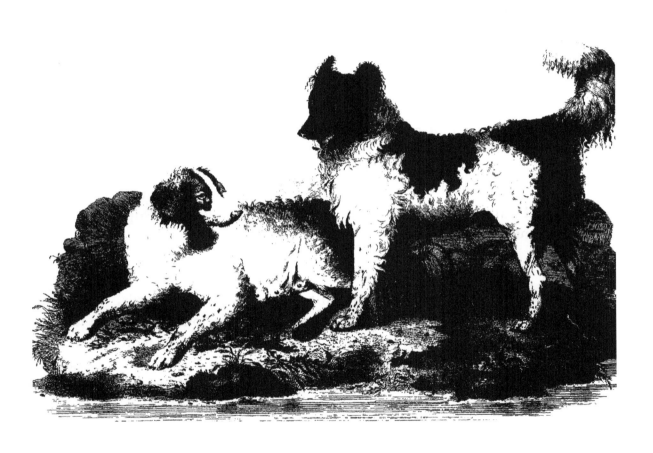

THE NEWFOUNDLAND DOG

London Pub by Syd Edwards Augt 1800

CANIS NATATOR.

THE NEWFOUNDLAND-DOG.

BEWICK'S Hist Quad. 326.

IS now universally admired and bred all over Europe, to nearly the extermination of many others. In this country we ought particularly to lament the rarity, if not the loss of the venerable Mastiff, for which England was once so famous, whose situation he now supplies, as a trusty and important guard to the person and property of his master.

The size, sagacity, and well known fidelity of these, deservedly entitle them to the most distinguished rank of all the canine race, although novelty should with the greatest caution be allowed to supersede long services and worth.

Their name is derived from the country of which they are supposed to be natives, but more probably introduced by the Spaniards, and great numbers have been imported into England, and various parts of the world, by vessels trading to and from Newfoundland, on board of which they are often kept, for the purpose of recovering any thing that has accidentally fallen into the sea, where they are not unfrequently lost, together with the object of their pursuit. It is the northern part of the island from which the true breed is brought; they are procured by the ships stationed there, and sent to the southern side, from whence they are transported to Europe and elsewhere.

" The settlers on the coasts of Newfoundland find them of the greatest
" service in bringing down the sledges loaded with wood, from the inte-

" nor parts of the country to the sea-shore; they tie or yoke several of
" them together, and three or four will draw two or three hundred
" weight with much ease, for several miles; when once taught, they re-
" quire no person to guide or drive them, and after having delivered their
" loading, return back to the place from whence they came, where they
" are rewarded with fish, of which they are very fond, both dried and
" fresh, and with which the country abounds from the great cod-fisheries
" carried on upon the coasts." But these are not the only kinds now to
be found in Newfoundland, for there are many others, probably carried
there by trading vessels, the natural consequence of an intercourse with
different nations.

The Dutch make use of various Dogs for the purpose of draft, and
place several a-breast in harness fastened to little barrows or carts loaded
with fish or merchandize, which they draw from Scheveling to the Hague,
and often return loaded even with men and boys*. Tradespeople in London also employ them in a somewhat similar manner; they are fastened
under their trucks or hand carts, where we often see them tugging like
little horses, with their tongues hanging out of their mouths almost sweep-
ing the ground; and were not the horse so common and so favourite
an animal amongst the English, great advantages might doubtless be
derived from their use in draft, which is exemplified in the more
northern nations, where horses are not so commonly met with.

In some parts of England, large Dogs are accustomed to drawing
water up from deep wells. Two of them usually work together within
a large wheel, to turn which their exertions are truly wonderful, barking
and disputing with each other for the greatest share of labour I was
much pleased with a scene of this kind in Hampshire, where one of the
Dogs, at intervals, quitted the wheel, and ran to the mouth of the well,
looking down to examine if the bucket was near the surface, then,

* Pratt's Gleanings

With us, the Newfoundland-dog seems to retain all its original purity, this climate being congenial to its nature and disposition; but when transported to a hot country, they gradually lose their vigour and beauty; one sent to Jamaica experienced a total change, by his waving coat falling off, and a very short smooth one succeeding, but upon his being taken to Canada, the hair resumed its former length and appearance; a similar circumstance is also related in Brown's History of Jamaica, as taking place with the sheep brought there by the Spaniards, the wool becoming short hair, but changing again upon their returning to their native place.

They sometimes grow to a very large size, but the general height is five or six and twenty inches, measuring from the top of the shoulder to the ground: large Dogs are sometimes higher behind than before, that is, from the highest part of the rump to the ground; but in speaking of their height, it ought to be considered as measured from the highest part of the shoulders to the ground. The length from the nose to the end of the tail is more than five feet. The most common colour is black and white, sometimes red and white, and more rarely of one colour, or black and white with tanned spots about the face.

The coat differs in various individuals, being in some short and curly, in others long and waving; the tail is large and bushy, and carried gracefully over the back; the ears, which it is customary to cut off, are short and pendulous; and the head in form strongly resembles that of a bear, from which they are often termed bear-headed.

The vulgar notion, that they are web-footed, will be found to be erroneous, the connecting part of the toes being similar to other large Dogs.

To the fowler on the sea-coasts their services are particularly necessary for fetching the wild fowl out of the water when shot, and their great strength and hardiness enable them to bear the severity of the weather, and fatigue of the sport, better than most others; nor are they deficient in scent, as many of them hunt tolerably well.

In swimming and diving, few equal, none excel them, and as their docility is so great, they most readily learn to fetch and carry small burdens in their mouths, of which employment they soon become fond; and these qualifications, added to the sincere attachment they shew to their masters, cause them to be highly esteemed

Among the many instances of their great sagacity, which might be adduced, those related by Mr. Bewick are well deserving our notice:

" During a severe storm, in the winter of 1789, a ship belonging to " Newcastle was lost near Yarmouth, and a Newfoundland-dog alone " escaped to the shore, bringing in his mouth the Captain's pocket-book; " he landed amidst a number of people who were assembled, several of " whom in vain endeavoured to take it from him The sagacious animal, " as if sensible of the importance of the charge, which in all probability " was delivered to him by his perishing master, at length leaped fawn- " ingly against the breast of a man who had attracted his notice amongst " the crowd, and delivered the book to him.

" The Dog immediately returned to the place where he had landed, " and watched with great attention for every thing that came from the " wrecked vessel, which he seized, and endeavoured to bring to land."

" A gentleman walking by the side of the river Tyne, and observing, " on the opposite side, a child fall into the water, gave notice to his " Dog, which immediately jumped in, swam over, and catching hold " of the child with its mouth, brought it safe to land."

To which the following may be added:

" A Newfoundland-dog, fighting with a Bull-dog at Bank-side near
" the Thames, appeared to be very hard put to it, and finding his adver-
" sary as obstinate as he was powerful, was observed to unite all his art
" and strength to draw the Bull-dog into the water, which he at length
" accomplished, and then very speedily drowned him."

" At the commencement of the gallant action which took place be-
" tween the Nymph and Cleopatra, there was a large Newfoundland Dog
" on board the former vessel, which the moment the firing began, ran
' from below deck, in spight of the efforts of the men to keep him
" down, and exhibited the most violent rage during the whole of the en-
" gagement. When the Cleopatra struck, he was among the foremost to
" board her, and there walked up and down the decks, seemingly con-
" scious of the victory he had gained."

When crossed with the Bull-dog, Wolf, or Mastiff, the produce becomes very furious and makes a useful Yard-dog, or Bear-dog, but should
rarely be trusted loose without a muzzle, as they are apt to seize without
discrimination horses, cattle, &c.

Crossed with the Setter they make an excellent sporting Dog for
marshy countries.

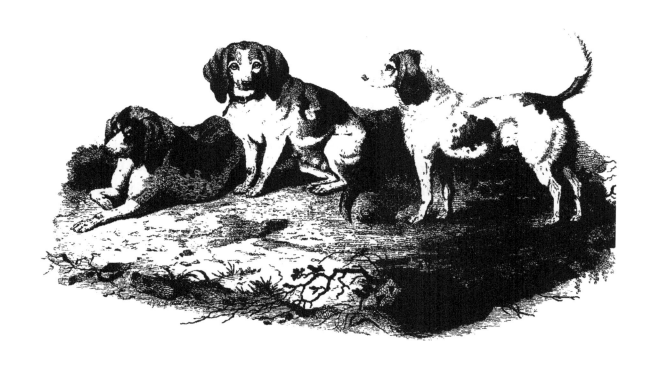

THE BEAGLE.

CANIS VENATICUS MINOR.

THE BEAGLE.

Canis venaticus minor —CHARLFTON
Canis minor celer, a Beagle —MERRET.
Beagle —BEWICK's Hist Quad

OF all the Hound tribe the Beagle is the least, and is used only for the purpose of hare-hunting. Their method of finding and pursuing their game is very similar to the Harrier, but they are far inferior in point of swiftness; yet to those sportsmen who hunt in a dry and inclosed country, where the coverts are not too large and strong, and who delight in unravelling the intricate mazes of the doubling hare, more than in the death, they afford no inconsiderable degree of amusement.

When the atmosphere is a little hazy, and the scent low, they catch it better than taller Dogs, spending their tongues freely in treble or tenor, and though more soft, yet not less melodious than the Harrier. But, as most sportsmen prefer the faster and stronger Dogs, these are by no means in such repute as formerly, a complete cry or pack of them being very rarely seen. They are now chiefly kept as finders to the Greyhounds in coursing, which purpose they answer extremely well, hence they are frequently called Finders.

The varieties are generally distinguished by the parts where they are bred, as, the Southern Beagle, bearing a strong resemblance to the slow deep-mouthed Southern Hound, but much smaller; the Northern Beagle, which is lighter formed, with shorter ears, and swifter· a cross breed between these two is esteemed preferable to either.

The Southern Beagles are smooth-haired, with long ears, and generally so loosely formed, that they cannot for a continuance be hunted in a heavy country without being crippled; besides which they have frequently some very great faults in a Hound, as crooked legs, tailing or lagging behind when they begin to tire, or are too small.

> " The pigmy brood in every furrow swims,
> " Moil'd in the cloggy clay panting they lag
> " Behind inglorious, or else shivering creep,
> " Benumb'd and faint, beneath the shelt'ring thorn "
>
> SOMERVILLE'S CHASE.

The Northern, which are commonly wire-haired, straiter limbed, and better formed in their shoulders and haunches, endure bad weather and long exercise with less inconvenience than the Southern.

They hunt hedge-rows, thread the brakes*, and muset † with the hare, with great spirit, but it is evident to the most common observer that neither of them are calculated to bear much fatigue.

Beagles, like other Hounds, are of various colours, and preferred as the fancy of the owner dictates   In height about twelve inches, and are hunted and treated in the same manner as the Harrier.

Mr. Pennant considers this Dog as the Agasæus of Oppian, and as a different variety from the Agasæus of Caius, for which it might be mistaken from the similitude of names, and says, " Oppian ‡ describes his as a " small kind of Dog peculiar to Great Britain," and then goes on, " Γυρον,

---

* To thread the brakes, in the language of the sportsman, is when the Dog examines with accuracy along every part of a hollow overgrown with briars, &c

† The muset of a hare is the hole in a hedge or enclosure, through which she passes, particularly when she relieves or goes to feed, and the dog is said to muset with her, when in the chase he pursues her through this hole instead of leaping over the hedge or going round about, by this means saving himself the trouble of recovering the scent. Generally called the muse, or mews

‡ Oppian, book 1 ver 419 to 526

" ασαρκότατον, λασιοτριχον, ομμασι νωθες. Curvum, macilentum, hispidum,
" oculis pigrum *Crooked, lean, rough, and slow in the eye**. What he
" adds afterwards still marks the difference more strongly; Ρινεσι δ᾿ αυτε
" μαλιϛα ωανεξοκος εϛιν αγασσευς†. Naribus autem longe præstantissimus
" est Agasseus‡. *But the Agasseus is most excellent in the nose.*

This is a truer description of our Terrier than the Beagle, particularly
that of the North, and doubtless his native original, as may be distinctly
traced in the rougher sorts: in this state it existed at the time of the pri-
mæval Britons, and by them was used for destroying the smaller vermin
and foxes, so detrimental to their hare parks§.

The British Blood-hound, or the large Southern-hound, bred with this,
would produce the several intermediate varieties of Staghound, Foxhound ‖,
Otterhound, Harrier, and Beagle, and by carefully preserving the smallest
offspring, but in make like the largest parent, would in process of time
form his exact miniature in the Beagle¶.

The term Beagle has been indiscriminately used by many for the Harrier and the Beagle, but is now wholly confined to the latter Are seldom
crossed with others unless to diminish their size, and are apt to challenge
any scent when hot, even that of birds.

* Whittaker says, *black-eyed.* See Terrier.
† Opp Cyneg lib 1 lin 473 476.
‡ Pennant's Brit Zool vol 1
§ Whittaker's History of Manchester, vol. 11
‖ To this class I consign the Agasæus of Caius, see Foxhound
¶ A learned and ingenious friend of mine to whom I am indebted for some curious trans-
lations and other valuable remarks, coincides with me in this opinion

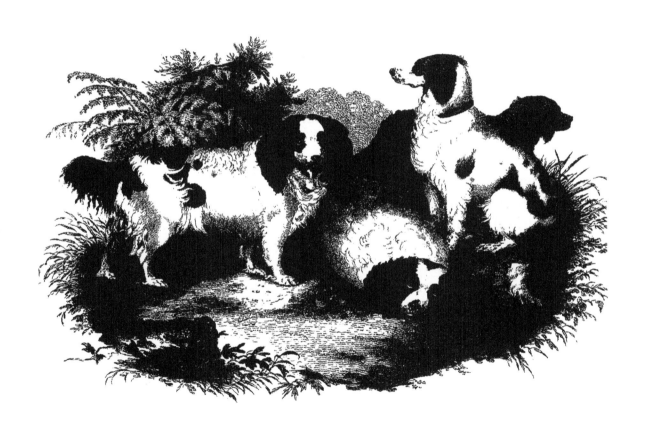

THE SPANIEL

CANIS HISPANIOLUS.

THE SPANIEL.

Canis Hispaniolus Agrarius, Land Spaniel —CHARLETON.
Canis Aviarius, seu Hispanicus Campestris.—RAII, 177·
Canis extrarius, Lin Syst
Canis Hispanicus, or Spanish Dog with hanging cars —ALDROV 561.
Epagneul or Spaniel, Buffon
Canis Hispaniolus, Spaniel —CAIUS.

THE name sufficiently indicates the country, to which this and the other sort of Spaniels owe their origin; and the Roman termination Hispaniolus or Spaniel, is a full demonstration of their Roman introducers*.

This was usually distinguished by the name of Land Spaniel, in contradistinction to Water Spaniel, and may be divided into two kinds, the Springing, Hawking Spaniel, or Starter, and the Cocker, or Cocking Spaniel; the first was used for springing the game when falconry was amongst the prevalent sports of this Island, and as it made one of the principal pursuits of our British ancestors, the chieftains maintained a considerable number of birds for that purpose. The discovery of the gun superseding the use of the falcon, the powers of the Dog were directed to the new acquisition; but his fleetness, wildness and courage, in quest of game, rendering him difficult to manage, a more useful kind was established, with shorter limbs and less speed; yet some of the true Springers still remain about London, but are rarely found in any other part of the

* Whittaker's Hist Manchester.

country, these are little different from the larger Spaniel or Setter, except in size; generally of a red, or red and white colour, thinly formed, ears rather short, long limbed, the coat waving and silky, the tail somewhat bushy, and seldom cut

Differing from this is the Cocker, esteemed for his compact form, having the head round, nose short, ears long and the larger the more admired, limbs short and strong, the coat more inclined to curl than the Springers, and longer, particularly on the tail, which is commonly truncated, colour liver and white, red, red and white, black and white, all liver colour, and sometimes black with tanned legs and muzzle.

From the great similarity of *some Cockers* to the Water Spaniel, both in person and disposition, little doubt can be entertained but *such are* derived from him and the Springer; some of the strongest of this kind are found in Sussex, and called Sussex Spaniels; another variety of Cocker much smaller is the Marlborough breed, kept by his Grace the Duke of Marlborough, these are red and white with very round heads, blunt noses, and highly valued by sportsmen.

Our unfortunate Monarch, Charles the First, was much attached to Spaniels, and had always some of his favourites about him; but these do not appear to have been the small black kind known by his name, but *Cockers*, as is evident from the pictures of Vandyke, and the print by Sir Robert Strange, after this master, of three of his children, in which they are introduced

The term Cocker, is taken from the woodcock, which they are taught to hunt, " but as all sportsmen know, it is singular, that no sporting Dog " will flush * woodcocks, till inured to the scent, and trained to the sport,

---

* Sportsmen say, flush a woodcock, spring a snipe, push a pheasant, and raise a partridge, when they are made to fly

SPANIEL.

" which they then pursue with vehemence and transport, though they
" hunt partridges and pheasants as it were by instinct, yet will hardly
" touch their bones when offered as food, but turn from them with ab-
" horrence, even when they are hungry, nor would a Mongrel Dog,
" though remarkable for finding that sort of game, but when offered to
" two Chinese Dogs, they devoured them most greedily, and licked the
" platter clean.   Now, that dogs should not be fond of the bones of such
" birds as they are not disposed to hunt is no wonder; but why they re-
" ject, and do not care to eat, their natural game is not so easily accounted
" for, since the end of hunting seems to be, that the chase pursued should
" be eaten.   Dogs again will not devour the more rancid water fowls,
" nor indeed the bones of any wild fowls; nor will they touch the fœtid
" bodies of birds that feed on offal and garbage; and there may be some-
" what of providential instinct in this circumstance of dislike; for vul-
" tures, and kites, and ravens, and crows, &c. were intended to be mess-
" mates with dogs over their carrion, and seem to be appointed by nature
" as fellow scavengers, to remove all cadaverous nuisances from the face
" of the earth*."   I may say the Spaniel possesses the soul of the chace,
madly pursues the object which cannot be reached by his limited powers,
triumphs when it tumbles from its aerial height, revels awhile till motion
ceases, but leaves it untasted to him who adds to his sport the gratification
of appetite.

Spaniels are used as Finders or Starters to the Greyhound, and pursue
the hare with the same impetuosity they do birds. Their beautiful coats,
their faithful dispositions, humble and insinuating manners, suavity and
obedience, even to servility, procure them universal favour, but the gunner
loves them for their intrinsic merit, bestows great pains on training them to
the gun, and when properly broke or educated, is amply repaid by their
services, being indefatigable in their exertions, beating the coverts, brakes,
and ditches, in pursuit of game; their tails carried downwards, perpetually
moving from side to side, and this motion, called feathering, becomes

* White's Hist Selbourne.

more rapid when they have caught the scent, eagerly following, with frequent whimpers, till it is disturbed, of which they give notice by repeated quests*, nor should they open at any other time; some sportsmen disapprove of their questing at all, as it spreads the alarm too far, therefore teach them to beat mute.

——————— " My Spaniels beat,
" Puzzling the entangled copse, and from the brake
" Push forth the whirring pheasant "

As it is the nature of these Dogs to put up all the game they find, good sportsmen are careful to keep them within gun shot, even in cover, and if it be extensive, gingles or bells are put on their collars, and the dog-call used if they beat too wide; those that are wild and riotous have one of the fore-legs buckled up, between the collar and the neck, till they are more steady. They pursue, without preference, the hare, pheasant, woodcock, snipe, partridge, quail, all water fowl, and most birds, are in general fond of the water, and easily taught to bring the game to their master. If taken out with Pointers, they should be led in a line while the Pointers are acting, lest by running into the game when the Pointers stand, they hurry them from their point, and make them unsteady; but they are useful to recover such wounded birds as take to running, especially pheasants They are more subject to certain diseases than other Dogs, as, loss of smell, swelling of the glands in the neck, which sometimes prevents their taking any sustenance till they die; disease on the ears like mange, called formicæ; and, lastly, to the mange itself, which is most destructive of all to their beauty and quiet.

They are sometimes crossed with the Pointer. Some of the puppies take after the Spaniel, and some after the Pointer, but have little to recommend them. For the training of them see Setter.

* Barking

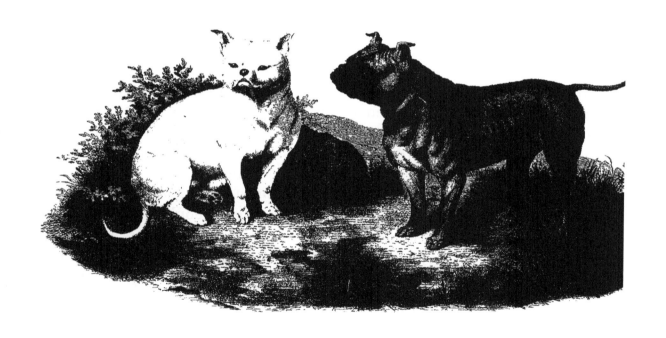

THE BULL DOG

CANIS PUGNAX.

THE BULL-DOG.

Le Dogue.—De Buffon, Hist Nat. V. p 249, t 43
Bull Dog —Penn Quad p. 242.

OF the various breeds of these animals observable in this country, not one possesses a stronger claim to being considered an original native of it than the Bull-dog; foreign nations having only obtained it by importation, and with them it is said to degenerate; which most satisfactorily accounts for the ambiguous character, and imperfect descriptions found in some continental authors, and the total silence of others on this head.

Among the few and earliest who have noticed it, is Buffon, who with admirable eloquence has written at great length on the various properties of many of the canine race, but has given us only a few unsatisfactory lines respecting this extraordinary branch of it.

He supposes, but with little apparent foundation, that the Shepherd's Dog brought into temperate climates, and among a people perfectly civilized, as those of Britain, France, and Germany, would, by mere influence of climate alone, lose his savage aspect, his erect ears, his rude thick long hair, and assume the figure of a Bull-dog.

Yet I am certain with respect to the Shepherds Dogs of this country, no such change ever does take place, even in the smallest degree; they remain unalterably the same, never partaking of the round head, the under-hanging jaw, and smooth coat of the Bull-dog

Some climates may have the power of altering the characters and properties of dogs, but in a temperate one like our own, we may observe
many distinct races, which, in spite of situation, retain, with very little or
no trouble, their peculiar and distinct qualities

Although Great Britain has always been famous for her fighting Dogs,
and long for her Bull-dogs, it does not appear from any accounts of them,
that the Bull-dog of the present day was the one intended, as the descriptions accord much better with the Mastiff, which was used for these purposes, and with which, as well as the Hound, it has been confounded by
later writers   The exact time this breed came into repute, or how produced, has hitherto eluded my most vigilant researches; that the Mastiff
was the Dog in estimation and use till within a short period, the writings
of many indubitably prove, even so late as the time of Gay, that accurate
observer of nature's varied forms and manners; and emphatically mentioned in his Fables of the Bull and the Mastiff, The Mastiff, &c.. nor is
it to be supposed, that had the Bull-dog and the Mastiff been as distinct as
at present, his critical judgment would have misplaced the one for the
other

I will venture to offer one conjecture on the subject, well aware that at
first sight it will not meet the concurrence of the amateur in Bull-dogs;
which is briefly, that about the time the Mastiff was common in England,
and after Gay, when bull and bear-baiting, with similar amusements,
was rapidly declining, especially among the great, the small Dutch Mastiff, or Pug-dog, was much in fashion, and probably by accident or design,
the mixture of these two produced the intermediate variety in question,
possessing the invincible courage of the one, with much of the form of
the other   Some objections may arise on account of the smallness of the
Pug, but it should be remembered, the diminutive size of many of these
creatures we are accustomed to see, is owing to their being bred as small
as possible for the purpose of lap-dogs, their original size being much
larger.

The Bull-dog is in height about eighteen inches, and weighs about thirty-six pounds; head round and full, muzzle short, ears small, in some the points turning down, in others perfectly erect, and such are called tulip-eared; chest wide, body round, with the limbs very muscular and strong; the tail thin and taper, curling over the back, or hanging down, termed tyger-tailed, rarely erected, except when the passions of the animal are aroused; the hide loose and thick, particularly about the neck; the hair short, the hind feet turned outwards, hocks rather approaching each other, which seems to obstruct their speed in running, but is admirably adapted to progressive motion when combating on their bellies; but the most striking character is the under-jaw almost uniformly projecting beyond the upper; for if the mouth is even they become shark headed, which is considered a bad point

The colours are black, salmon, fallow, brindled, and white, with these variously pied; the fallow, salmon, and brindled with black muzzles, are deemed the most genuine breeds, and the white to possess most action: there is a strong general resemblance between a brindled Bull-dog and the striped Hyæna

The diversion of bull-baiting, for which this dog is almost exclusively used, is much less common than formerly, and it is not improbable that it may, together with him, be known to posterity but by name It is supposed by some to be of Roman origin, by others, " to have taken its rise " together with bull-running from some of the tenures of the manor and " castle of Tutbury in Staffordshire, as appears by the charter granted to the " king of the minstrels, who amused the crowd attendant on the hospitality " of the ancient Earls and Dukes of Lancaster, by John of Gaunt.

" In the reign of Henry the Fourth, the Prior of Tutbury gave the " minstrels who came to matin on the feast of the Assumption of the " Blessed Virgin, a bull to be taken on this side the river Dove, otherwise " the prior paid them forty pence.

" This custom continued with divers alterations after the reformation.
" On the 16th of August 1680, the minstrels (as annually) met in a body
" at the house of the bailiff, when they were joined by the steward of the
" manor (then belonging to the Earl of Devonshire) a sermon was preached
" to them by the vicar of the kirk, on the origin and excellence of music,
" each minstrel afterwards paying him one penny; they then adjourned
" to the banqueting-hall, where a dinner was provided, after which the
" bull was demanded of the prior; the victim was turned out to be taken,
" with his horns cut off, his ears cropped, and his tail curtailed to the
" very stump, his body besmeared over with soap, and his nostrils filled
" with pepper, to irritate and increase his rage and fury.

" Thus savagely equipped, the bull was let loose, a solemn proclama-
" tion was announced by the steward, that none were to approach him
" nearer than forty feet, nor to hinder the minstrels, but to attend to
" their own safety. The minstrels were to take this enraged bull, before
" sun-set, on this side the river Dove; which if they could not do, and the
" bull escaped them into Derbyshire, he still remained the property of
" the lord of the manor.

" It was seldom possible to take the bull fairly; but if they held him so
" long as to cut off some of his hair, he was then brought to the market-
" cross, or bull-ring, in the middle of the street and mart, and there
" baited, after which the minstrels were entitled to have him.

" Hence originated the rustic sport called bull-running and bull-bait-
" ing, which has continually been gaining ground till of very late years;
" the above custom is ultimately abolished by the noble owner of the
" castle, and will probably have the desired effect upon those similar
" diversions of bull-baiting practised in many country towns at that season
" of the year called the wake*."

* Plot's Nat Hist Staff chap x

" The custom of baiting the bull at Stamford, in Lincolnshire, had its
" rise from this occasion. In the time of King John, William, Earl of
" Warren, and Lord of the Town of Stamford, standing upon the castle
" walls, saw two bulls fighting for a cow, in the adjoining meadow, till
" the butcher's Dogs being roused therewith, pursued one of the bulls
" (madded with noise and multitude) quite through the town. Which
" sight so pleased the Earl, that he gave the castle meadows, where first
" the bull's duel began, for a common to the butchers of the town, after
" the first grass was mowed or eaten, on condition that they should find a
" mad bull the day six weeks before Christmas Day, for the continuance
" of the sport every year; which custom is still observed, and occasioned
" the proverb (used among the people and others, in that county and
" elsewhere) *As mad as the baiting-bull of Stamford* *.

At Abergavenny, in Monmouthshire, famous for this sport, it was usual
to bait one or two bulls on St. Crispin's Day, the chain was dragged about
the streets, to give the shopkeepers, and others, previous notice thereof;
the most vicious bulls were selected for that purpose, and their breed of
Dogs were justly celebrated.

The idea that the flesh of the bull is rendered more tender from being
baited, was perhaps another cause for the frequency of this sport; and I
believe there is still an act of parliament unrepealed, forbidding, under
pains and penalties, the selling of bull beef unless it had been baited,
or a lighted candle be kept burning during the time of sale, to prevent
imposition.

The properties of the British Bull-dog are matchless courage and perseverance, even to death; to develop the difficulties to which he is exposed
by the amateur, presuming on this courage and perseverance, is not a
pleasing task, but is imposed on me by the nature of the subject.

---

* Butcher's Survey of Stamford, p. 40.

Bred for the combat, and delighting in it, he evinces against an un-
equal adversary, invincible courage; roused by injury, or led on by his
master, he attacks the most powerful animal, and rushes upon it without
the slightest indication of fear; disdaining stratagem, he bravely assails the
enemy in front, the bull, the buffalo, or bear, and if successful fixes his
powerful jaws on the nose, bringing the head to the ground pins it there,
destitute of the power of resistance, till in loud roarings his superiority is
confessed   The smaller animals, as rats, mice, &c he rarely regards.

When the bull is baited, he is secured by a strong rope, or a chain,
about twenty feet long, to a ring and stake fixed in the ground, the other
end being fastened about his neck, a circle is formed round him by the
spectators, and one or two dogs only are allowed to give him battle at
once; they are no sooner loosed within the ring, than they run at and
endeavour to seize the bull by the nose, if they succeed and pin him, he
is unable to retaliate the injury, but, bellowing with revenge and pain,
lowers his big forehead to the earth

On the other hand, the bull with watchful gloomy aspect waits the approach of the dogs, with his head downwards, receiving them on his
horns, throws them alternately sprawling into the air, or suddenly lifting it
up, lets them pass between his legs, and on their return, tosses or tramples
them under his feet.

In matches fought for prizes the Dogs are first prepared, to enable them
to bear the fatigue should the battle be lasting; if fat, they are reduced to
moderate leanness by purgatives or fasting, regularly taken out for exercise, and suffered sometimes to go into the water, particularly in warm
weather   Twelve or fourteen days are considered as sufficient time for this
preparation, during which they are fed with raspings, crusts of bread, or
biscuits mixed with water or broth, and for the few last days with boiled
milk, but little flesh is given them, and that always dressed   On the day

appointed for fighting they receive no food, or only a bit of toasted bread, so they come to battle empty and hard in flesh.

These matches at the bull are of two kinds, one which is termed the *turn-loose match*, when two dogs are turned loose at the same time, and the one that continues the attack longest wins the prize; no person being allowed to interfere with the Dogs till one of them ceases to fight. The other, called the *let-go match*, in which they are let go alternately, each Dog having a person who acts as second, running a part of the way with him towards the bull, and is ready to catch him up as soon as possible after having reached the bull's nose. The Dog that runs the greatest number of times at him is declared victor. There is also a person in this latter match who seconds the bull, and gives him notice of the Dogs being loosed by the word halloo, and both Dogs are run from the same spot.

Bulls which are accustomed to be baited on these occasions are called game bulls; these seldom attempt to injure the populace, are admirably dextrous in defending themselves, and round knobs of wood are fastened on the tips of their horns to prevent their goring the Dogs.

In the *turn-loose match*, when much fatigued with fighting and falls, some lay awhile on the spot they are thrown to, and having recovered their breath a little, renew the combat with fresh vigour. this habit gives them advantage over the opponent, and is deemed one of their valuable properties. After the battle is over, if the weather be cold, they are kept warm till somewhat restored, otherwise they are in danger of perishing. The punishment the Dogs undergo, and their returning to the contest, are considered as the test of their courage; and as the object in this case is not to pin the bull, the tusks are sometimes filed down to prevent their fixing on him, which renders them liable to be broken, and not unfrequently the jaw also.

" Magnaque taurorum fracturi colla Britanni* "

" And British Dogs subdue the stoutest bulls."

* Claudian de Laud Stilichonis, lib. iii line 301.

In baiting the bear this breed is preferred to all others; and here the love of the combat, impelled by blind rage on the one part, opposed on the other by ill-directed strength, urged by necessity; the headlong attack, the tardy defence, together with the grotesque ferocious character of the combatants, afford a scene truly risible. In this amusement, next to the bull-bait, the amateur delights*

A ring is fixed in a wall, and to it a rope a few feet long is appended, and made fast to the collar of the bear; in a contrary direction, fastened to the collar also, another is held by his keeper. The Dog assails with a scream, and is answered by a muttering growl; the bear-keeper giving the halloo, pulls the rope, assisting the bear to rise on his hind-legs, who places his back against the wall, parrying off the Dog, and raising his nose in the air to prevent its being seized. The Dog, in leaping at the nose, is grasped round the neck or body, thrown to the ground, and hugged with violence, breathing is suspended, the tongue swelled and hung out; the eyes reddened, forced from their sockets; the blood vessels of the throat and mouth ruptured. From this terrible embrace he is disengaged by his owner dragging him off by the tail or legs, the bear never persisting in his hold. Notwithstanding this dreadful reception, he immediately returns to the combat undaunted. In the number of these returns his master discovers his bottom, and boasts his game.

Sometimes the bear adopts another mode with his headlong adversary. A young Dog being loosed, rashly precipitates himself against him; this, coolly observing, Bruin dexterously steps aside, and applying a blow with his paw to increase his velocity, dashes his head against the wall with the utmost violence, making him suffer severely for his temerity. A good handler prevents this, by running his Dog sideways to the bear, and parallel to the wall.

If the Dog succeeds in seizing the bear, he becomes furious, and tears him with his teeth and claws. When long exasperated, he has recourse

---

* This sport is not of modern date. See Mastiff

to stratagem, which for that time, and perhaps for ever, rids him of his enemy. Having thrown the Dog, and made a hole with his teeth, he forces, by means not easily discovered, a quantity of air betwixt the skin and flesh; it immediately swells, spreading wider, and without instant assistance the Dog seldom recovers: several incisions should be made with a sharp pointed knife, the air should be pressed out, and the parts dressed. This is a curious fact, well known to the amateur. To handle a Dog well, is to take him quickly but gently from the bear. The winning Dog is he that runs oftenest, fighting fair, that is at the head, not at the legs, which, if he prefers seizing, he is not permitted to run again.

The ass, I believe, is baited in London only, and seldom even there. This patient object of oppression here exhibits a more spirited character; he becomes alert and formidable; on being attacked, he brays vehemently; defending himself dexterously with his fore-legs, he proves almost as serious an antagonist as the bull, often laying his adversary prostrate, and stunned on the ground, with broken bones.

In fighting with each other the mode of attack is entirely altered. They now lay hold wherever they can, and from the muscular powers of jaw, retain their hold an amazing time; they acquire a knowledge of the tenderest points, and aim chiefly at these, the base of the ear, the shoulder, joint, elbow, brisket, and particularly the legs; these the old and crafty fighter endeavours his utmost to seize, which his antagonist labours to prevent, by keeping them much under his belly, his breast almost touching the ground, presenting his head and neck only: thus continuing the fight lying or standing till one fights no longer, or turns away, which, if but to take breath, he loses the battle and the prize. At other times they are fought by making a scratch on the ground, near which, after the turning away of either, they are placed, and over it are run alternately at each other till one refuses, the other going over wins. They are generally matched by weight.

It has been discovered, that by rubbing over the head, neck, legs, and shoulders of a Dog with nauseous or acrimonious ingredients, another

Dog will not seize him, nor will he, if well-bred, run away, but take all the punishment the other gives without ever biting. When this is detected, the person playing the trick forfeits the prize.

Although the wounds the Bull-dog inflicts are not severe, yet by his unsubdued and obstinate courage he will in general conquer any other of an equal or even superior size. It is probable that the teeth, not acting in immediate opposition from the great projection of the under jaw, may prevent his tearing like other fighting Dogs; but the principal reason is his retaining to his uttermost the same hold, and though successful in overpowering, not proceeding to destroy his enemy; it is probable too, this apparent deformity, the elongation of the under jaw, facilitates his seizing objects above him in combating, as the nose of the bull, bear, &c.

Destitute of scent, incapable of tuition, slow and sluggish in his manner, loose and irregular in his gait, in his pacific moments apparently inoffensive and stupid, sulky in the eye, and averse to action; but roused by noise, and easily wrought to a pitch of madness; seizing whatever presents or opposes him; nor is he deterred from the furious assault by lacerated limbs or broken bones.

Of his admirable courage, the sportsman has of late discovered how he may avail himself. Many have been sent to India, the island of Hispaniola, and the borders of the Black River Jamaica, where they are used in the hunt; the wild cattle or buffalo being brought to bay by fleeter dogs, and fear keeping aloof the pack, the Bull-dog, ever brave and unappalled, rushes to the attack, and, aided by the hunter, closes the scene.

They may be *over bred*, that is to deep game but loss of action, suffering pain without resistance.

They are properly crossed with any other Dog where courage is the requisite.

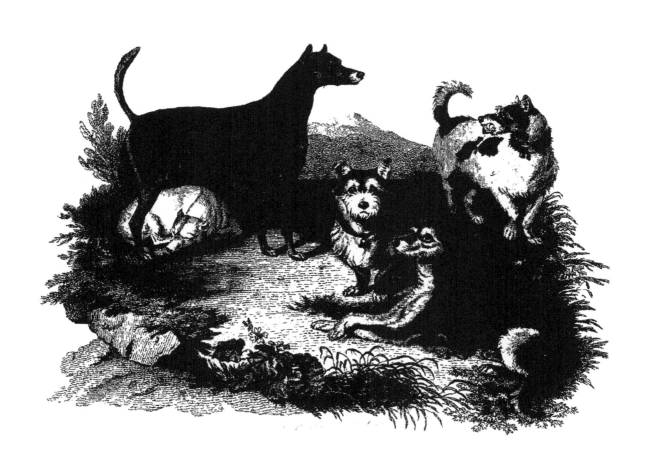

THE TERRIER.

THE TERRIER.

Canis Vertagus, Terrier.—LINNÆUS
Canis Terrarius, Terrier.—CHARLETON.
Canis Terrarius, Terrare.—CAIUS
Terrier.—BEWICK'S QUAD
Le Basset a jambes torses, Le Basset a jambes droites.—BUFFON
Canis Vertagus.—RAII SYN. ANIM

SO called from earthing or entering holes after its game. From the evidence of Oppian's* Poems, he appears to be an original native of this island.

" A small bold breed, and steady to the game,
" Next claims the tribute of peculiar fame,
" Trained by the tribes on Britain's wildest shore,
" Thence they their title of Agasses † bore
" Small as the race that, useless to their lord,
" Bask on the hearth, and beg about the board,
" Crook-limbed, and black-eyed, all their frame appears
" Flanked with no flesh, and bristled rough with hairs,
" But shod each foot with hardest claws is seen,
" Its kind protection on the beaten green,
" Fenced is each jaw with closest teeth around,
" And death sits instant on th' inflicted wound
" Far o'er the rest he quests the secret prey,
" And sees each track wide opening to his ray
" Far o'er the rest he feels each scent that blows
" Court the live nerve, and thrill along the nose "

* Oppian lived in the days of Severus, A D. 194.
† A Gast or a Gass (as Kist, the same word is also Kis) signifies merely the Dog
Whit Hist. Manch.

Linnæus says, it was introduced upon the Continent, so late as the reign of Frederic the First. It is doubtless the Vertagus or Tumbler of Rau and others*. Rau says, it used stratagem in taking its prey, some say tumbling and playing till it came near enough to seize. This supposed quality, natural to all the cat race, when applied to the Dog I consider as mere fable; but it has led to a strange error, after-naturalists having from this concluded, a Dog of valuable and extraordinary properties was entirely lost.

The most distinct varieties are, the crooked-legged and straight-legged; their colours generally black with tanned legs and muzzle, a spot of the same colour over each eye though they are sometimes reddish fallow, or white and pied. The white kind have been in request of late years. The ears are short, some erect, others pendulous, these and part of the tail are usually cut off; some rough and some smooth-haired many sportsmen prefer the wire-haired, supposing them harder biters, but experience shews this is not always the case. Much of the variety in the Terrier arises from his being a small Dog, and often bred for mere fancy.

The Terrier is querulous, fretful and irascible, high-spirited and alert when brought into action; if he has not unsubdued perseverance like the Bull-dog, he has rapidity of attack, managed with art, and sustained with spirit, it is not what he will bear, but what he will inflict. his action protects himself, and his bite carries death to his opponent. he dashes into the hole of the fox, drives him from its recesses, or tears him to pieces in his strong hold; and he forces the reluctant stubborn badger into light. As his courage is great, so is his genius extensive: he will trace with the Fox-hound, hunt with the Beagle, find for the Greyhound, or beat with the Spaniel. Of wild cats, martens, polecats, weasels, and rats, he is the vigilant and determined enemy he drives the otter from the rocky clefts on the banks of rivers, nor declines the combat in a new element.

* The Vertagus of Caius. See Lurcher.

The straight-legged Terrier is hunted with the Fox-hounds in England, but when the fox goes to earth it is not a desirable quality that he should seize or destroy him, as this would put an end to the pleasure of the chase; the Terrier, when sent in after him, drives him out, or to a corner of the hole; to ensure his chambering the ground should be struck above to oblige him; the yearning of the Dog will direct the digger, who in digging down should place the spade between the Dog and the fox, least there should be more in the hole than one. if these precautions are not used, he will bolt, or else remain in the widest part of the burrow, where the angles meet, that when dug to, he may retire to which chamber he pleases: this is generally the resource of those foxes or badgers who have once escaped. A small bell or gingles may be fastened to the collar of the Dog, which assist in alarming the fox, and making him chamber sooner; and also in directing those who dig with more certainty. So great is the Terrier's perseverance, that some have been known to remain in the earth for days together, until both the fox and themselves have been nearly starved to death.

The badger hunt is practised in moonlight nights, when they are abroad in search of food, and the ultimatum is to sack the badger. The holes previously found, two persons or more should join: care must be taken to reach the den or burrow without noise, availing themselves of the wind; the Dogs kept close to the sportsmen, and silent to prevent alarm; all the holes being carefully stopped but one, the sack with a running string must be put into this, and one left to watch; then the sport begins.

Those that guide the Terriers go to the extremity of the badger's known range and slip the Dogs, each sportsman should be prepared with a long stick, to the end of which should be affixed a barbed hook. The Terriers soon find, and immediately commence the attack; it is, however, seldom but in the earth that the Terrier will instantly fasten. The badger makes home, and maintains a running fight. Should the sportsmen overtake the chase, which they may easily do if swift of foot, they encourage the Terriers, and try to catch him with their hooks; but let them beware, the bite of the badger enraged is not only severe, but difficult to heal; should the badger reach home, the hole-keeper must exert all his dexterity to secure him, and exclude the Terriers, whose ardour is increased as they approach the hole. If the sack is forced, and the badger earths, the Terriers must be kept back, for on them depends the fortune of the chase. Select your most determined Terrier, and keep him up. If the hole is without many windings, fix a string, not too strong, to the hind legs of your terrier that is to run, joining them together, put a rope through this, and running it double keep the two ends in your hand, and run him; he will meet a rough reception; if he does not fix, but retires and yearns, draw immediately and change him for another; run them alternately; if your Terriers have been fleshed they are sure to assail; if these fail run the favourite, and you will have the pleasure of seeing the badger dragged to light.

When trained to kill rats, acquaint them intimately with the ferret who shares the sport. The ferret put into the rats hole drives them out; the Dog watches, and as they bolt, springs upon them with incredible dexterity and dispatches them at a gripe, never missing his aim or mistaking the ferret for a rat.

In Scotland the use of the Terrier is to kill; and here they breed a fierce race; so great is their courage they will attack and destroy the largest foxes with which that country abounds, following them into the chasms of rocks, where they often perish together.

If the breed is known and sure, the Terrier should not be entered till twelve or fifteen months old. A badger or fox may be muzzled and put into a hole, and an old Dog or two sent in after him, the young ones held near to listen and see them act; the old Dogs may then be taken up, and the young ones encouraged to fight, which if well-bred they will soon do, a cub-fox or badger may be procured for them to kill, for if they are bitten hard when too young they seldom turn out well. Cats are particularly injurious to puppies.

Badgers are commonly caught for baiting, and killed for their skins, fat, or flesh; the hams dried are esteemed excellent.

Although Terriers are used for baiting badgers and fighting one with another, yet few will bear the severity of either; a cross of the Bull-dog is often added to give them *stay*. The badger, though harmless in most respects, is a dreadful opponent to the Terrier, nor could he be overcome but by the craftiness of the assailant, who attacks him under the breast and belly.

From the fiercest of the Terrier breed and the Bull-dog is produced a good fighting Dog; crossed with the Blood-hound, or Southern-hound, a good Fox-hound; with the Fox-hound an Otter-hound; and with the Greyhound a Lurcher.

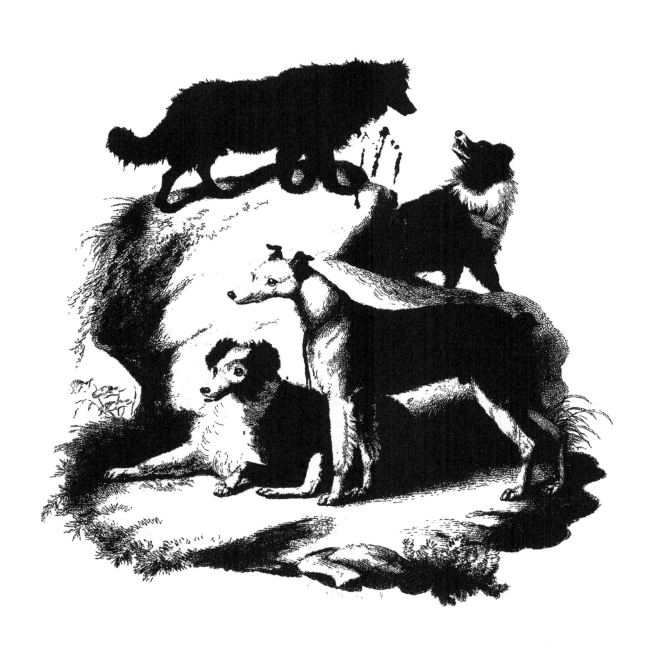

THE SHEPHERDS DOG
AND
THE CUR

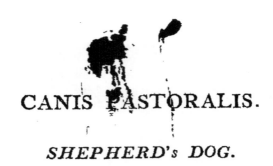

CANIS PASTORALIS.

SHEPHERD's DOG.

Shepherd's Dog.—BEWICK.
Le Chien de Bergher —BUFFON
Canis Pastoralis —CAIUS

THE Shepherd's Dog seems so universally disseminated, that it would not be easy to name the country to which it belongs. The useful obtains a universality, denied to that which is sought for only by the idle for amusement, or by the great for pomp or pleasure. To restrain the flock on the pathless plain, and recal the bold straggler, to obey the commands of an humble and unlettered master, were not likely to procure distinction and a name; yet his properties, peculiar to himself and essential to the wandering shepherd, must have early spread his breed wherever the pastoral life prevailed.

Buffon considers this the parent stock from which the other varieties branch out, and has given a very extraordinary genealogical table, shewing the mode of ramification. This hypothesis makes the Shepherd's Dog a native of northern climes; and sending him to Ireland he becomes a Greyhound of prodigious size, with a long muzzle; but in Britain a Bull-dog of small stature, with a muzzle short to deformity; in Siberia and Lapland he becomes small and savage; he is a Bull-dog in Britain without scent, but then again he is a Blood-hound in Britain with a very fine scent and large pendulous ears, merely because men are civilized.

To me his ingenious system appears false on the following considerations. A mixture of a pure race can only produce a pure race, for although size and make may be cultivated from particular individuals, yet the difference in make will be slight, and the size and instincts have early limits

But admitting that two dissimilar individuals would produce the Bull-dog and Irish Greyhound, in crossing these together the mongrel should tend towards the parent stock; instead of which, says Buffon, it becomes a mastiff, that is, a Dog of a different make and different instincts, both to his immediate parents and to his original ancestor; and this too in a climate where the Shepherd's Dog is in perfection

The Dog, carnivorous by nature wherever he is found in a wild state, is generally a hunter, using the nose, associating in packs, and satiating himself with blood; but from the Count's system he should always be a Shepherd's Dog, harmless to the harmless, and careful for the weak.

In islands first noticed by civilized man, Dogs excessively dissimilar have been found in use, and perfect in their powers, as the Blood-hound, Terrier, and Mastiff in Britain

The Dog is as much attended to now in all his varied properties, and as much crossed as ever; and if one stock has produced the numerous rare varieties, it should follow of course that new kinds possessing new properties would continually arise; yet no such effect takes place, and no mongrels, when perpetuated by long breeding, have any valuable qualities differing from the parent stock

Variety of climate, subjugation to man, and liability to his caprice, if it has produced such striking varieties in the Dog, might and should have equally affected the Horse, who is as much attended to, and equally the object of caprice and fashion; yet difference of size seems the only alteration that takes place, his general external appearance remains fixed.

In all countries where the various races are said to have arisen from degeneration or cultivation, the Shepherd's Dog retains, in company of the Bull-dog, Irish Greyhound, Beagle, and Spaniel, his simple appearance, his sharp muzzle, his flowing coat, his pensive melancholy aspect, and his useful yet harmless exertions.

Attending to cattle by the eye without using the scent, and without offering injury; associating together in packs, and by the scent tracing large animals and devouring them for food; attending to the inhabitants of the air, and rejecting for food that which they assist to destroy; pursuing animals under ground, or launching after them in the watery element; imply the possession of such contrary properties as could not be procured from one pure origin by culture merely. Nature seems to have confounded nothing, and I think it is agreeable to her general laws, that an animal destined to act so conspicuous a part, to exert such different powers, to extend the authority or increase the pleasure of man, was originally produced in distinct varieties, if not species. How numerous were the original kinds it would not now be easy to determine; the whim and caprice of man doubtless has produced many mongrel races, that time has given a permanency to; still the higher qualities seem to remain very distinct.

To the position of there being of the Dog different original species, one objection may be made; how, as they freely mix, have they remained distinct? To this I answer, it has been indubitably proved, that the fox, jackal, wolf, and domestic Dog will mix, and the offspring reproduce, yet no confusion has taken place in the desert; general character would present a bar, and instincts, disposition, and habits, confine them to different districts; and finally, man, finding the value of his acquisition, would early direct his attention to keep the various races distinct.

The Count de Buffon was fond of theories and systems, and he has formed some very extraordinary ones to account for the grand phenomena of nature. Of a daring and sublime genius, a varied, acute, and perspicuous reasoner, an elegant and animated writer, he has made specious what was doubtful, and emblazoned his opinions with beautiful imagery, and all the charms of language   Had a writer of less favoured powers formed the hypothesis on Dogs, it must have met with immediate opposition, and ever been considered as visionary.

The Shepherd's Dog is about fourteen inches high, nose sharp, ears half pricked, coat moderately long, somewhat waving, thick about the neck and haunches, tail bushy with an inclination upwards towards the point, seldom erected, colour all black, black with tanned muzzle and feet, or black with a white ring round the neck and white feet; most have one and some two dew claws, of all Dogs he seems the most thoughtful, most pensive, and most melancholy

His properties, peculiar to himself, are retaining in memory a command given, which he will execute at an after period on simply recalling it by a hint; his proceeding at *signal* to any given point, and, though in the heat and hurry of action, conforming himself strictly to command, and obedient to the wave of the hand, a wonderful attachment to the place of his birth and education; retaining his love for the memory of a lost master even to death, and often refusing his services to another

To the Shepherd who guides his flocks on mountainous regions or extensive plains his services are invaluable; he will proceed to great distances, down one hill he will cross a valley and ascend another; here out of reach of the voice he will obey the wave of the hand; if from distance the hand becomes invisible, he will perform the same figure on a large scale his master describes by moving on his station; he will proceed over a mountain's top, and, surrounding the flock, bring them into view, which when he has done, he stops to observe his master's intentions   in this manner he saves him traversing many a weary mile, and performs services that without his aid could not be achieved.   When a few Sheep for any purpose are selected from the flock, he then exerts all his ability, and an arduous task he has to perform.   Sheep on mountainous regions are swift as Roes. If well taught he never approaches too nigh, but hovering round presents himself wherever his presence is necessary. He surrounds them with rapidity, prompts them to their proper course, restrains their ardour to his master's pace, punishes with a sharp and sudden turn the bold adventurer that would escape, observes his ground in the line of march, and exerts his attention if there is danger of escape If the whole burst away in a body, he flies before for fear of separating them, makes half circles and meets them in front; sometimes by a rapid attack on the whole, at others on the most forward, whom he carefully marks, still keeping them in a body, he completely overpowers, and reconducts them to his master.

That Dog is in the highest degree perfect, who will in this manner conduct the smallest number of Sheep in a body. There are Dogs who will manage four; selected and put under their care, they will alone and unassisted conduct them to their master's dwelling, although at the distance of some miles.

On the wild, the sole companion of his master, he conceives for him the most lively affection, resenting any injury offered him if but in jest; without prompting he will bite the heels or fly at the neck of the assailant, nor is he deterred by menaced blows. None dare approach when his master sleeps; he is then on the watch, and is often known to awake him when accidents happen or danger appears that he cannot avert. Employed only on real business, he is not playful or frolicsome, but sedate and pensive, in action he is alert according to necessity, vigilant, active, and sincere; he gazes on the flock scattered over the mountains with an attentive eye, and considers them as under his controul; he never offers injury, attacks but to restrain, and pursues but to guide. The best kinds run perfectly silent.

When Sheep are flocked in narrow bounds they may be for hours entrusted to his management; he may be taught those bounds, and will of himself restrain them to its limits.

The Count de Buffon has asserted that he is born perfect in his instincts, and requires no training. The evidence of a single Shepherd would have confuted him in this I will assert that no Dog requires so much. The great object is to make him run wide from the flock, and appear only at the points where he is wanted; when they fly away to teach him to make half circles, and meet them suddenly in front, by this means he fatigues the sheep less, whether in driving or gathering them together. No assistance is got from running him with a trained Dog, as this only prompts a heedless attack. A young Dog, when first tried, runs amid the flock, dispersing them without any apparent design, or selecting one and pursuing it, his education proceeds entirely from his master, and, I must observe, few arrive at the first perfection

As it is unlikely this work should meet the Shepherd's eye,

" Whose thoughts fond science never taught to stray,"

I forbear to subjoin instruction for training; I besides consider that necessity makes them adepts, and their being indolent to a proverb prompts to this point their exertions. To shew how far this Dog's powers may be cultivated, I copy the following anecdote from Dr Anderson.

" Of the sagacity of Dogs many instances might be adduced ; but none
" that I have ever met with can equal the following instance of the saga-
" city of a Shepherd's Dog. The owner himself having been hanged some
" years ago for sheep-stealing, the following fact, among others, respect-
" ing the Dog, was authenticated by evidence on his trial When the
" man intended to steal any sheep, he did not do it himself, but detached
" his Dog to perform the business. With this view, under pretençe of
" looking at the sheep, with an intention to purchase them, he went
" through the flock with his Dog at his feet, to whom he secretly gave a
" signal so as to let him know the individuals he wanted, to the number
" of perhaps ten or twelve, out of a flock of some hundreds; he then went
" away, and from a distance of several miles, sent back the Dog by him-

" self in the night time, who picked out the individual sheep that had been
" pointed out to him, separated them from the flock, and drove them be-
" fore him by himself, for the distance of ten or twelve miles, till he came
" up with his master, to whom he delivered his charge."

Few instances occur in which the Shepherd's Dog offers to hunt, and those that take to it are easily deterred. They are crossed with some mongrel breeds, and produce a good Dog for driving cattle.

CANIS DEGENER. CHARLTON.

THE DROVER's DOG, OR CUR *.

The Cur —BEWICK's Quad

THE Drover's Dog stands highei on his legs, is larger and fiercer than the Shepherd's Dog; coloui black, brindled oi grizzled, with generally a white neck, and some white on the face and legs, sharp nose, ears half pricked or pendulous; coat mostly long, rough, and matted, particularly about the haunches, giving him a ragged appearance; many are *self tailed* †.

Inferior agents are never used, but when affairs of little importance are to be carried on; it would appear to be even a waste of animal intelligence to employ a Dog of a superior mind simply to urge tame cattle forward in a beaten path, highei properties being unnecessary, chance has produced the Diovei's Dog, from piobably a commixture of Shepherd's Dog, Lurchei, Mastiff or Dane; his restless manner, shuffling gait, incessant barking, vagabond appearance, and perpetual return and reference to his master, bespeak him incapable of any great design, or regulai chain of action, and mark him complete mongrel; being of little value, his place may easily be supplied in other countries by other mongrels, and he appears peculiar to England, being rarely found even in Scotland. He is useful to the farmer or grazier, for watching or driving their cattle, and to the

* Vide lower figure on the plate.   † Whelped without a tail

drover and butcher for driving cattle and sheep to slaughter; he is sagacious, fond of employment, and active; if a drove is huddled together so as
to retard their progress, he dashes amongst and separates them till they
form a line and travel more commodiously; if a sheep is refractory and
runs wild, he soon overtakes and seizing him by the foreleg or ear, pulls
him to the ground. The bull or ox he forces into obedience by keen bites
on the heels or tail, and most dexterously avoids their kicks. He knows his
master's grounds, and is a rigid centinel on duty, never suffering them to
break their bounds, or strangers to enter. He shakes the intruding hog by
the ear, and obliges him to quit the territories. He bears blows and kicks
with much philosophy, and notwithstanding the nonchalance of his manner, is very cunning, a great poacher, and destructive to hares and rabbits.

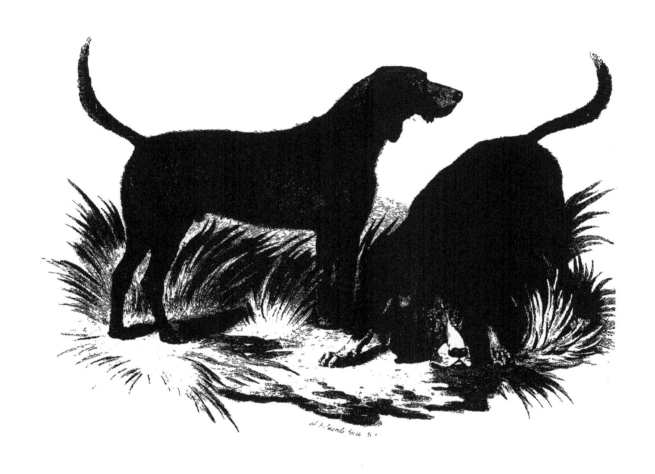

THE BLACK HOUND

London Pub by and Edwards & Charles Street Queen Film Jan 1803

BRITISH BLOOD-HOUND.

Blood-hound.—BEWICK's Quad.
Canis sanguinarius, seu furum deprehensor, a Blood-hound.—RAII
Canis sanguinarius, Blud-hund.—CAIUS.
Canis Scoticus, Blood-hound.—KERR.
Blood-hound —SHAW's Quad.
Canis sanguinarius, Blood-hound, or Sleuth-hound —PENNANT's Quad.

THE Bloodhound is about twenty seven inches high, of a strong, compact, and muscular form; the face rather narrow, stern, and intelligent, nostrils wide and large; lips pendulous; ears large, broad at the base and narrowing to the tip; tail strong, but not bushy; voice extremely loud and sonorous. But what most distinguishes this kind, is their uniform colour, a reddish tan, gradually darkening on the upper part, with a mixture of black on the back, becoming lighter on the lower parts and extremities. One of the Dogs I saw, had a little white on the face, but this was not usual with that breed. Mr. Pennant mentions their having a black spot over each eye: this was not the case with either of those I made the drawing from.

When the nobler animals are long bred in pure blood, added to valuable properties, whose uses are intrinsic, and whose application is extensive, all the finer traits come into view; they obtain a bold stamp from nature that none mistake; while the philosopher examines with attention, he perceives a mind, an instinctive intelligence, in these her elder offspring; a pure character and genuine value.

Such is the impression made on viewing the Blood-hound.   His stern forehead, his eyes piercing and firm, his massive and capacious nose, long pendulous ears, his large yet compact figure, made for strength and action, his uniform colour, a voice only inferior to the Lion's roar, and in unison to the deep toned horn, bespeak him the companion to the ancient chieftain, the hunter of old   I am not here to discuss, whether we have gained or not by adoption or crossing, but I must lament the scarcity and probable loss of this grand race , and hope our sovereign, or some of our nobility, will yet form a pack, and give them perpetuity   to a royal assemblage of men and horses, what an accompaniment !

" To scour the wild,
" And sweep the morning dew "

The antiquary preserves in museums, from all corroding time, the bust that modern art can imitate, the character of the oldest manuscript the pen or graver can trace, and translation perpetuate whatever it contains useful or elegant, but if a race of animals is lost, human power cannot restore them.

The British Blood-hound, though not so swift as the Fox-hound, is superior in fleetness to the Talbot-hound, does not dwell so long on the scent, nor throw himself on his haunches to give mouth ; but having discovered his object, goes gaily on, giving tongue as he runs.   There is no doubt he was originally the only Dog used to trace the game by the scent in this country.   The manner of the ancient hunt was not at all that now practised   the game was found and surrounded in its haunts , when roused it was shot by the arrow, or wounded by the spear, if in this state it escaped, the Blood-hound traced, and the Mastiff or hunter killed it ; but there was nothing similar to our chase. When the game run in view, it was pursued by a Dog swift of foot, probably the Irish Wolf-dog, or Shagged Scotch Grey-hound   The chase, as now practised, was doubtless derived to our ancestors from the continent, and packs were formed at no very remote period   The Dog that hunted was then required swift to head the horses. It would readily occur to the hunter to give a cross of the Terrier, who has a most delicate scent, to procure speed, and hence our present Fox-hound. The great peculiarity of the Blood-hound is his tracing any thing that has lost blood; from this his name is derived, and to this and tracing the deer-stealers his education is directed. When about a year old, a deer recently killed is dragged to some distance, and he is put upon the trail with a staunch old Hound, and rewarded at the end of each hunt with part to eat: when perfect in this lesson, the shoes of a man are rubbed with deer's blood, and he makes a circuit of a mile or more, renewing the blood occasionally; the circuit is made more wide and intricate, as the Dog becomes more experienced: his last lesson is to hunt a man dry foot, which he will soon atchieve with the assistance of an old Dog, and when he succeeds in this singly, his education is complete, as with a little practice he will hunt man or any animal.

The learned and philosophic Boyle, in his Essays of Effluvia, c. 4. instances, the high perfection the Blood-hound was made to arrive at, when his powers were attentively cultivated. " A person of quality, to whom " I am near allied, related to me, that to make trial whether a young " Blood-hound was well instructed (or as the huntsmen call it made) he " caused one of his servants, who had not killed, or so much as touched " any of his deer, to walk to a country town, four miles off, and then to a " market town three miles distant from thence ; which done, this noble-" man did, a competent while after, put the Blood-hound upon the scent " of the man, and caused him to be followed by a servant or two, the mas-" ter himself thinking it also fit to go after them to see the event; which " was, that the Dog, without ever seeing the man he was to pursue, fol-" lowed him by the scent to the above mentioned places, notwithstanding " the multitude of travellers that had occasion to cross it, and when the " Blood-hound came to the chief market town, he passed through the " streets without taking notice of any of the people there, and left not till " he had gone to the house, where the man he sought rested himself, to

" the wonder of those that followed him. The particulars of this narra-
" tive, the nobleman's wife, a person of great veracity, that happened to be
" with him when the trial was made, confirmed to me."

On the borders of England and Scotland, while the countries waged
fierce wars, the moral principle was in a manner extinct, and private rob-
beries were sanctioned as military incursions; what in war under their
leaders the feudal tenant seized by force of arms, in peace he stole under
cover of the night, and drove his prize in darkness far within his own districts, or secured it in fastnesses here the Blood-hound was of wonderful
use, as he would trace either the thief or cattle *.

And while the barbarous clans of the north, under petty chiefs, were perpetually engaged in civil broils, the vanquished, who fled from the sanguinary conflict, were often hunted from cave to cave by the Hound, and
slaughtered in cold blood. In those popular tales and heroic ballads, which
recite the chivalrous exploits of the brave Wallace, they are oftened men-

* " Soon the sagacious brute, his curling tail
" Flourish'd in air, low bending plies around
" His busy nose, the steaming vapour snuffs
" Inquisitive, nor leaves one turf untry'd,
" Till conscious of the recent stains, his heart
" Beats quick, his snuffling nose, his active tail,
" Attest his joy, then with deep-op'ning mouth,
" That makes the welkin tremble, he proclaims
" Th' audacious felon foot by foot he marks
" His winding way, while all the list'ning crowd
" Applaud his reas'nings O'er the wat'ry foid,
" Dry sandy heath, and stony barren hills;
" O'er beaten paths with men and beasts distain'd
" Unerring he pursues, till at the cot
" Arriv'd, and seizing by his guilty throat
" The caitiff vile, redeems the captive prey,
" So exquisitely delicate his sense !"

tioned: and the hero of his country, when his followers separated to avoid or distract the pursuit of numbers, was frequently obliged to take curious precautions, against the sure scent of the hound.

Of his race, nearly extinct, a few preserved in pure blood are in the possession of Thomas Astle, Esq. and his family; and to his kindness I am indebted for leave to make the drawing from which the figure is given, and for the account of the mode in which they are trained, probably of very remote antiquity.

I give the following account of a hunt as related to me by Mr. Astle. It having been discovered that two deer were killed in Needwood Forest, Mr. Astle immediately let out the dogs, and, putting them on the foot of the thieves, commenced the chace; on the first alarm of the cry, they dropped one of the deer, and after a considerable time the two haunches of the other deer, and then the remaining parts; still finding the pursuit close on them, they threw aside their coats and waistcoats, and were seen at nearly a mile distant, running with the greatest swiftness quite stripped; in a little time one was in combat with a dog, when he drew them off.

The deer stealers however found out a mode of escaping; they strewed pepper on their steps, which the dogs snuffing up, were for some time prevented from finding the scent.

As a watch dog, none can exceed the blood-hound; being strong and fierce; in the country if the alarm was given too late for detection he would still pursue the felons footsteps. I hope this being more generally known, may bring his estimable talents into notice, and prevent the loss of a valuable race.

Mr Bewick says, there was a law in Scotland, that whoever denied entrance to one of these Dogs in pursuit of stolen goods, should be deemed an accessary.

CANIS ANTARCTICUS.

THE DINGO, OR DOG OF NEW SOUTH WALES.

Dog of New South Wales,—GOVERNOR PHILLIPS's Voyage
Dingo, Australatian Dog, or Dog of New South Wales.—SHAW's Quad

HE adds to the general appearance of the fox and wolf a considerable degree of elegance; is near two feet high; coat short, somewhat rough about the neck and haunches; muzzle pointed; eyes piercing; ears short and erect; tail bushy and hanging downwards; of a pile brown colour, darkening on the upper parts and lighter beneath the muzzle; cheeks, breast, insides of the legs and feet, nearly white.

The naturalist and philosopher have remarked, that the various forms of being approximate, and from the higher to the lower afford a beautiful gradation; like the long drawn shadows of a summer evening, which by joining the varied objects of the landscape leave no part unfinished, but form of its disjointed masses a perfect and distinct whole. There is a charm by long acceptance attached to the idea, that it is like profanely intruding on hallowed ground to suggest any thing which might dissipate it; yet the inquirer after truth accepts it with great reserve; he sees nature never confuses; and in innumerable orders of existence, perceives betwixt each a powerful barrier or impassible gulph, whether in the mute and irrational tribes, the superior brute instinct, or in man, who rears his sublime front to the heavens, perceives and reasons. But although the idea of shading in the picture be rejected, the philosophic observer who enters the temple of nature, feels and acknowledges that no space is void; the gradation appears necessary, and is complete; a perfect and solemn order reigns there, sustained by the great parent,

> ' Who can the finny tribes, though mute,
> " To Cygnets dying accents raise "

I have already observed, that where animals approach nearest, no intermixture takes place in the desert; particularly between the wolf, the fox, or jackall. The dog is easily tamed, nor readily quits man for liberty and his native wilds The wolf, fox, and jackal, are nearly irreclaimable. The wolf is solitary, and differs much from the dog in his external appearance; the shoulders approach near in front, and produce a narrow chest; his eye unsettled and frequently changing; his tushes, strong in the insertion, open his otherwise tapering muzzle broad above the nostrils; he never barks but howls, his gait is solemn, yet irregular; when enraged against his own species, he continues the attack to death, his aspect is savage, and his grin horrid.

The dog loves to associate with his kind; he possesses gaiety, and gracefulness, a steady eye, and playful countenance; his chest is broad, and his gait firm, he is capable of attachment, even to the loss of his own life; if roused to assail his own species, he only proceeds to conquer, and would not kill, unless urged on by man. When the dog howls he laments; but he constantly barks, and in this manner often expresses his joy, or his attachment to his master.

Individuals of the Antarctick dog have been brought into this country and kept in our menageries; in this state of confinement they are pretty docile, but have not shewn any attachment to their keepers; our knowledge of them being very imperfect, I had some queries, through the

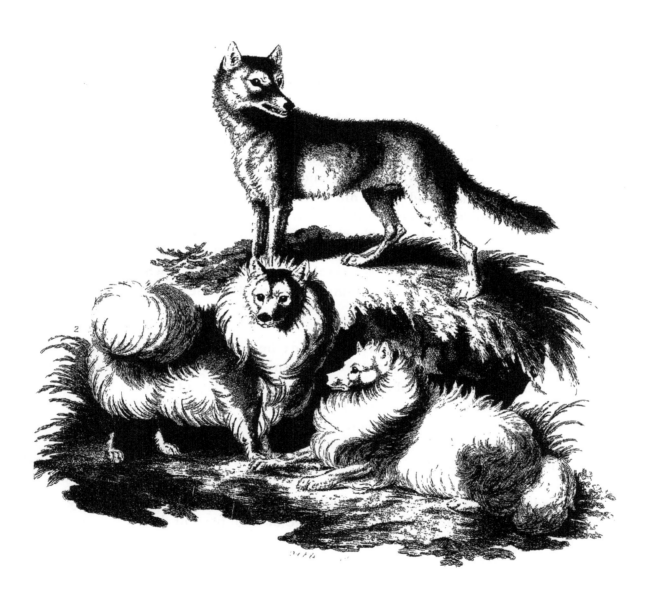

medium of a friend, put to Major George Johnstone, of the New South Wales corps, who has resided there thirteen years, and the information thus obtained I give in his own words.

" They chiefly reside about the cove heads, and under the rocks, near
" Sydney; have been found to litter in hollow trees; and are frequently
" seen in all parts of the country that has been explored; they hunt singly,
" nor are they ever seen in parties; they do not bark, but make a long
" dismal howl; not easily domesticated, but have been made to follow a
" master, though, whenever opportunity offers, will seize any fowl or ani-
" mal that comes in their way; their common food, the kangaroo, and
" kangaroo rats."   The time of gestation is unknown.

When the figure, which was copied from life, is attentively examined, and the few known particulars of their character and economy considered, I think it doubtful, whether he is a Dog or a variety of the Wolf; without venturing my private opinion on such slight materials, I shall leave it open for the observation of future naturalists.

CANIS POMERANUS.

POMERANIAN, OR FOX DOG.

Le Chien Loup —Buffon.
Canis Pomeranus —Kerr

HEAD broad towards the neck and narrowing to the muzzle; ears short, pointed, and erect; about eighteen inches high; is distinguished by his long, thick, and rather erect coat, forming a ruff around the neck, but short on the head and ears; of a pale fallow colour, lightest on the lower parts, some are white, some black, but few spotted; the tail large and bushy, curled in a ring on the rump; instances are few of short coated ones

He is known in England by the name of Fox Dog, probably from his bearing some resemblance to a fox about the head, but by authors who describe him as native of Pomerania, more properly termed Pomeranian Dog

He is of little value as a House Dog, being noisy, artful, and quarrelsome; cowardly, petulant, and deceitful, snappish and dangerous to children, and in other respects without useful properties. He is very common in Holland, and there named Kees; has been used by the caricaturists, partisans of the house of Orange in opposition to the Pug, to ridicule the patriots in their late political disputes. There is a peculiarity in his coat;

his hair, particularly the ruff around his neck, is not formed of hairs that describe the line of beauty, or serpentine line, but is simply a semicircle, which by inclining the same way in large masses, give him a very beautiful appearance. Although his attachment is very weak, yet is he difficult to be stolen. The largest are used for draft in Holland.

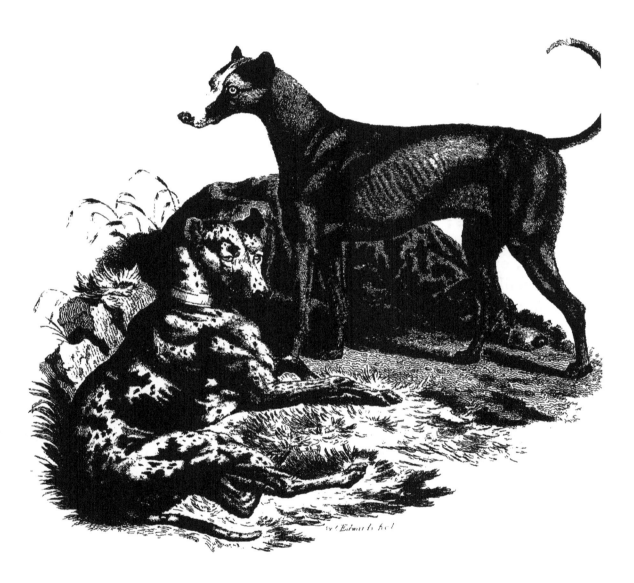

THE DANISH DOG.

Pub. Nov 1. 1799 by Syd Edwards, N 11 Charles Street Queen Ann.

THE DANISH DOG.

Le Grand Danois.—BUFFON.

THE Dane is about twenty-eight inches high, some will reach thirty-one inches; in form he is between the Greyhound and Mastiff; head straight, muzzle rather pointed, ears short, half pendulous, usually cropped, eyes in some white, in others half white or yellow; chest deep, belly small, legs straight and strong, tail thin and wiry, in some curled over the rump, in others more straight; colour sandy red or pale fallow, with often a blaze of white on the face; a beautiful variety, called the Harlequin Dane, has a finely marbled coat, with large and small spots of black, grey, liver colour, or sandy red, upon a white ground; the two former have often tan-coloured spots about the face and legs.

The grand figure, bold muscular action, and elegant carriage of the Dane, would recommend him to notice, had he no useful properties; and thence we find him honoured in adding to the pomp of the noble or wealthy, before whose carriages he trots or gallops in a fine style, not noisy, but of approved dignity becoming his intrepid character, he keeps his state in silence; that he is obliged to be muzzled to prevent his attacking his own species, or other domestic animals, adds much to the effect, as it supposes power, and gives an idea of protection. The common Coach Dog is an humble attendant of the servants and horses, the Dane appears the escort of his lord, bold and ready in his defence, and the harbinger of his approach. I certainly think no equipage can have arrived at its acme of grandeur until a couple of Harlequin Danes precede the pomp. I do not know at what time he was introduced into England, nor whether he was ever used here for any but the above purpose.

The British Sportsman rejects his services, because he does not add art to force, and is unfit for modern refinement; but with the hunter of old, who traversed the trackless Scandinavia, he would procure honourable distinction; and, fearless as his fearless master, who exposed his person to imminent peril in the chase, would attack the larger animals, nor could it be till a modern æra that he was disused, as we find him frequently figured in the paintings of Snyders and Rubens, and in the prints of Ridenger; there, swift, powerful, and fierce, we see him rush to the combat, and instantly close with the wolf, boar, or stag, nor have I observed that he is represented at bay. But when the dark woody forest, retired before cultivation and inclosed pasture, and the sanguinary, ferocious, or solitary tribes fled the populous haunt, the Dane then became a subject of peace, and a servant of shew; yet even now he might be useful to the gamekeeper to pull down wounded deer, but he must be kept in subjection, as he attacks sheep with deadly fury.

He is courageous and fearless, he makes love to the combat, and rejoices in the battle; that he is capable too of affection, and attaches himself to a master, we have proof of in Lord Cadogan's Dane, figured in the Tapestry of the siege of Bochain at Blenheim, who attended his master in all the actions of the gallant Marlborough, and returned in safety.

Whether the Orientals use him in the Tiger hunt I do not know, but in the East they term him the Tiger Dog.

Theie is a variety of the Dane figured by Buffon, a small Dog not known in England.

The Dane, where beauty, stiength, and courage are the requisites, might be ciossed with the Mastiff, Irish Greyhound, or Newfoundland Dog; but as a lover of nature, fiom his fine figure, his couiage, his speed, his perseverance, I should like to see his iace perpetuated in pure blood.

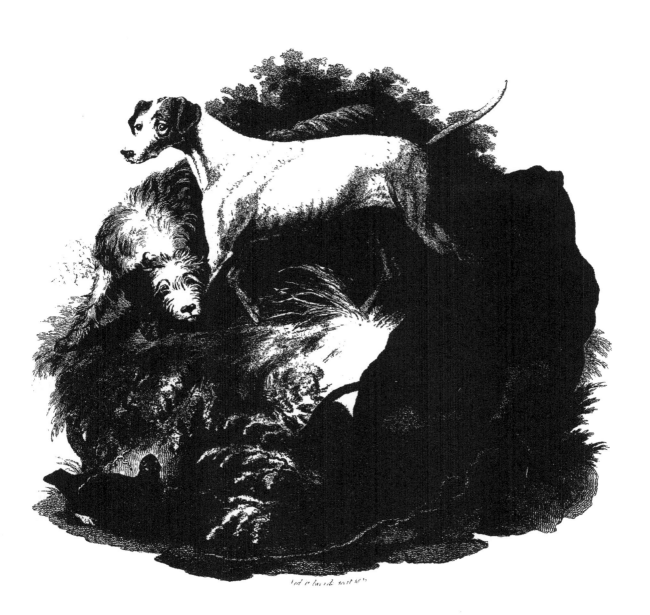

THE POINTER

CANIS AVICULARIS.

THE POINTER.

Canis Avicularis —LINN.
The Spanish Pointer —BEWICK

THE Spanish Pointer is a heavy loose made Dog, about twenty-two inches high, bearing no small resemblance to the Slow Southern Hound ; head large, indented between the eyes ; lips large and pendulous ; ears thin, loose, and hanging down, of a moderate length ; coat short and smooth ; colour dark brown, or liver colour, liver colour and white, red and white, black, black and white, sometimes tanned about the face and eyes, often thickly speckled with small spots on a white ground ; the tail thin, smooth, and wiry; frequently dew claws upon the hind legs the hind feet often turning a little outwards.

The Spanish Pointer was introduced to this country by a Portugal Merchant, at a very modern period, and was first used by an old reduced Baron, of the name of Bichell, who lived in Norfolk, and could shoot flying ; indeed he seems to have lived by his gun, as the game he killed was sold in the London market. This valuable acquisition from the Continent was wholly unknown to our ancestors, together with the art of shooting flying ; but so fond are we become of this most elegant of the field sports, that we now excel all others in the use of the gun, and in the breeding and training of the Dog.

The Spanish Pointer possesses in a high degree the sense of scenting, so that he very rarely or never goes by his game when in pursuit of it; requires very little training to make him staunch, most of them standing the first time they meet with game, and it is no uncommon circumstance for puppies of three months old to stand at poultry, rabbits, and even cats; but as they grow old they are apt to get idle, and often go over their ground on a trot instead of galloping, and from their loose make and slowness of foot, when hunted a few seasons, soon tire, have recourse to cunning, and in company let the younger and fleeter dogs beat wide the fields, while they do little more than back them, or else make false points; they then become useless but for hunting singly with a sportsman who is not able or not inclined to follow the faster Dogs.

The sportsman, aware of these disadvantages, has improved the breed by selecting the lightest and gayest individuals, and by judicious crosses with the Fox-Hound to procure courage and fleetness. From the great attention thus paid has resulted the present elegant Dog, of valuable and extensive properties, differing much from the original parent, but with some diminution of his instinctive powers   He may be thus described . Light, strong, well-formed, and very active; about twenty-two inches high , head small and straight , lips and ears small, short, and thin ; coat short and smooth, commonly spotted or fleched upon a white ground, sometimes wholly white; tail thin and wiry, except when crossed with the Setter or Fox-Hound, then a little brushed

This Dog possesses great gaiety and courage, travels in a grand manner, quarters his ground with great rapidity, and scents with acuteness ; gallops with his haunches rather under him, his head and tail up, of strength to endure any fatigue, and an invincible spirit ; but with these qualifications he has concomitant disadvantages ; his high spirit and eagerness for the sport, render him untractable and extremely difficult of education; his impatience in company subjects him to a desire to be foremost in the points, and not give time for the sportsman to come up, to run in upon the game, particularly down wind; but if these faults can be overcome in training, if he can be made staunch in standing, drawing, and backing, and to stop at the voice, or token of the hand, to come in to the charge, rate, or call, to wait till he is cast off again, never to leave or break the field without the sportsman, to bring the game when shot without breaking it, never to pursue what escapes, and to take water, he is highly esteemed; and those who arrive at such perfection, in this country, bring amazing prices.

That this perfection may be attained, it is necessary to begin in a proper manner; the usual method is ill calculated to ensure success, and success seldom attends it. The young Dog is suffered to run wild without the smallest tuition, till he is twelve months old; in a state nearly ungovernable he is put into the hands of some breaker or game-keeper, who, if the Dog does not train himself, treats him with such severity, that he is commonly returned entirely ruined. If the following method is attentively pursued, I have proved it will be attended with compleat success. Procure your puppy from parents well formed and of a staunch breed; teach him by gentle means, as early as possible, to fetch and carry, to come in when called, and to bear confinement; these early lessons acquired will save an infinite deal of trouble afterwards; he should be kept constantly chained, and only loosed for exercise, or to receive his lessons, which should be twice a day.

He may next be practised in the common way, with a bit of bread; when he is hungry, take hold of his collar, and throw a piece before him, and when he offers to snatch it, call out, *Take heed, softly,* and hold him some time before you give the word, *go, seize,* or *lay hold*. Should he be impatient to take it before the signal is given, correct him gently This must be repeated, till he will stop for the word without being held, nor should he ever be permitted to take the food offered without first taking heed, to confirm his being in perfect command.

He may, when strong enough, be taken into the field, and suffered to range about almost wherever he pleases, but encourage him to cross and range before you. Take him to one end of the field, turn your back to the hedge, and cross in an oblique line to the other, directing him with your voice and hand to accompany or go before you ; repeat this, by turning round and walking in a similar direction to the other side ; this may be continued, and if he performs tolerably well, he should be caressed Although he should be ever so unruly, he must only be corrected by the voice, or other gentle means, for if he happens to be of a timid disposition, he will be terrified by rough treatment, and never range out again. Should he accidentally fall upon game, he will probably put it up and pursue ; this must also be suffered at first ; and if he runs out of the field, he must be brought back by calling his name, and cautioning him, *gently, come back.* Larks often puzzle a young Dog, but if you caution him by the words, *Ware Lark,* he will cease to pursue them, and his eagerness will soon abate when he finds he pursues in vain.

Most young Dogs are subject to rake, that is, to hunt with their noses close to the ground, of which habit they should be broke expeditiously and effectually, if possible ; for if a Dog rakes, following the birds by the foot, he will never make a good Pointer, nor find half so much game as the Dog who carries his head high ; therefore if you perceive your Dog following a bird by the foot down wind, call to him by his name, and give the words, *Hold up* ; on being checked he will become agitated and uneasy, going first on one side, and then on the other, till the wind brings him the scent of the birds. If he repeats this a few times, and is regularly checked, he will take the wind himself and hunt with his nose up; but the best method of curing a Dog of this fault, is hunting him on moors, or where the ground is uneven, and covered with low furze, heath, and brambles; these prevent his holding his head down, and oblige him to range higher. On moors the best Dogs are trained. If this is not attainable, and you are under the necessity of breaking him on level land, or in a local situation, recourse must be had to the puzzle peg; the construction of this is simple; it consists of a piece of oak or deal inch board, a foot in length, and an inch and a half in breadth; tapering a little to one end; at the broadest, are two holes running longitudinally, through which the collar of the Dog is put, and the whole is buckled round his neck, the piece of wood being projected beyond his nose, is then fastened with a piece of leather thong, passing through his mouth, at the back of the long teeth of the lower jaw, so as to tie the peg under his chin; by these means the peg advancing seven or eight inches beyond his nose, the Dog is prevented from putting his head to the ground and raking.

The next lesson, is to bring him to stand, and the most stubborn or wild may be made steady by perseverance, if their natural instinct is good. To accomplish this object and bring the Dog to game, fry some small pieces of bread in hog's laid, with the dung of partridges or pheasants if it can be procured, and having made him take heed, and seize a piece or two, at home, take the bread in a little bag into the field, and place the pieces in several different places, marking the spot with little cleft pickets of wood, which will be more easily distinguished by putting small pieces of cards in the niches. The Dog may then be cast off, and by giving him the wind, conducted to the places where the bread lies; when he gets the scent, if he approach too near, and seem eager to fall upon it, call out, in a menacing tone, *take heed*, and correct him with a whip, he will soon comprehend what is required of him, and will stand; when he understands this lesson, take a gun charged with powder only, and walking gently round the bread, fire the gun off instead of crying seize, and let him eat the bread; on repeating this, walk round the bread several times, before you fire, making him wait till his impatience is conquered, and he will keep his points till the signal is given.

When this is carefully practised he may be entered at game; and for this purpose, if a partridge cannot easily be procured, take a game chicken of a brown colour, and place it in the corner of a room; he may be encouraged to take notice of it, and cautioned from seizing it, as in former lessons; the legs of the bird being tied, a pistol loaded with powder only should be fired at it, and he may be suffered to bring it to you, which he should do by gentle means, and be encouraged when he will do it without injuring the fowl.

It may next be taken into the field; and fastened by a string and peg to the ground, cast the Dog off, and by giving him the wind, he will soon hit upon the fowl; if he stands well, fire off the gun at some little distance, go up, unloose the peg, and make him bring it to you, always observing if he bites it hard to check him with moderation. To any objection that may be urged against a chicken, I have to observe, in the field there can be no confusion take place, and the Dog will always seek after and prefer the strongest game; every good sportsman must have noticed, that some of the oldest and best Dogs will stand to domestic fowls in a hedge, when they accidentally meet with them, as staunch as to a pheasant, to which nature has nearly allied them; observing this, led me to the useful mode I recommend. A rabbit may be used after the same manner as a fowl to break him to hares.

Having acquired these preliminary instructions, he may be safely hunted where there are partridges; by giving him the wind, he will probably behave well; but should he run in, and raise the birds, you must return to the live fowl, or bread, till he is more steady; should he remain at his point till you are up with him, encourage him to draw on the birds by calling, *Hie on boy*, softly, and when you want him to stop, *To ho*, and by always repeating this, he will become acquainted with the words and hunt with care, stop, and go on, as you direct him.

If a Dog has not been early taught obedience, it is found difficult to make him stand, till you are up with him; recourse then must be had to the strong collar, in order to check him completely. The collar consists of a strong and rather broad leather strap, stuck through with three rows of small nails, the points of which penetrate a little way through the surface of the inside; a strong piece of leather is then sewed over the heads of the nails on the outside, to prevent their starting back when the points are pressed against, a ring is fastened to each end of the collar, because if buckled in the common way, it would continually wound the neck of the Dog; these rings are fastened loosely together by a piece of string, so that the collar may hang about the neck, and to this string may be appended one end of the trash cord; which is a piece of rope of about twenty fathoms in length, and this he must drag after him; when he stands, make up to him, and warning him to take heed, lay hold of the cord; should he attempt to run in, or bark, when the birds rise, check him smartly by pulling the rope, which presses the points of the nails against his neck, at the same time calling sharply, *take heed*; by repeating this a few times, he will become afraid to commit the same fault ; if the strong collar is thought too severe, the trash cord may be fastened to his own collar, and used in a similar manner, or it may be pegged down by a peg fastened to the trailing end. Calling him by name is highly proper when he is corrected, as he will understand better when he it spoken to in company.

By these methods, although he may be accomplished in his business, it will still be necessary to hunt him singly. At first a few birds may be killed upon the ground to him, and he may be made to bring them to your foot, and lastly he may be hunted in company with a staunch old Dog, the observance of whose manner will now be of the greatest service to him. When the old Dog makes a point, if the young one is at some distance from him and inattentive, he must be called to by name, and the stop words given him *To ho* ; if he does not stop and back to the old Dog, but run up to the point, and hurry him from it, he should be called in, and chastised smartly, repeating his name ; he must not be let go, but make him lie still and try to shame him of his fault ; in a little time after he should be called to you, and the matter made up by patting him on the head and side, speaking kindly to him lest he become timid and refuse to hunt again the rest of the day. By perseverance and practice, he will amply repay the labour of the breaker

There are other varieties of the Pointer ; as the Russian ; in size and form like the Spanish ; coat not unlike a drover's Dog, rough and shaggy, rough about the eyes and bearded, colour like the Spanish, but often grizzle and white ; they differ in some being more rough than others ; this is probably a cross between the Spanish Pointer and the Barbet, or rough water Dog ; he has an excellent nose, sagacious, tractable, and easily made staunch ; endures fatigue tolerably well ; takes water readily, and is not incommoded by the most cold and wet weather; he will frequently prefer laying in a hole formed in the snow to the shelter of his kennel; his whole frame is loose, and his travelling slow.

The Ladies Pointer is a variety too diminutive for use.

In the possession of the late Mr. Beckford, was a beautiful drawing, after Titian, of two Pointers, which, according to Mr. Beckford, were the same as those used in France; narrow head, fine muzzle, and light limbs; are very staunch and fleet; one of the Dogs has a feathered tail; but from Scotland, where the French Dog is not at all uncommon, I am assured that he is a perfect model of the Spanish, only smaller and firmer in his make; and I am at a loss to conceive, what Dog the Spanish Pointer could be crossed with, to produce the sharp muzzle and feathered tail, unless with the English Fox Hound. The contiguity of France to Spain, a champaign country, and plenty of game, would also be a presumption that in the Spanish Pointer all the properties wanting might be found; but this may be easily ascertained by any sportsman who visits France, and also whether a cross from them would improve our breed.

There is a circumstance worthy of notice in Pointers, that some of them have a deep fissure in the centre of the nose, which completely divides the nostrils; such are termed *double nosed*, and supposed to possess the power of scenting better than others.

Pointers stand truly to partridges, pheasants, grouse, ptarmigans, snipes, woodcocks, quails, landrails; to hares and rabbits. They are not fond of taking water, or entering coverts. When hunted in woodlands, the bell collar should be put on their neck, to give notice when they stand.

Shooting flying to the Pointer is certainly the most elegant of the field sports; the talent of the man is called into action as well as the Dog, for the flying game must be killed at a certain distance, and the time must be marked to half a second, or it escapes The rapidity of its flight, the alarm at its rising, the exertion to meet the instant, the agitation of the Dog, and the momentary anxiety for success, certainly to the lover of the sport give an electric shock of animal pleasure inexpressibly grateful , it is enjoyed too at a season, when the frame relaxed by the summer suns, wants the cooler breeze of September to prepare it for heavy damps and the severity of winter

He who follows the Dog regularly through autumn, may bid defiance to the fogs of December and the frost of January, and brave the dripping covert or the stormy moor. Nothing can be more beautiful than to see a brace of well-trained Dogs, ranging, backing, or standing, all agitation and tremblingly alive to every effluvia the gale brings, examining all its variations, until the sought for odour meets the olfactory organs, and then, as if by some irresistible power struck motionless, appear like a piece of petrified stone They commonly stop with one leg up, and some indicate the particular game found, or the distance they are from it, by their manner of pointing; some drop gently down on their bellies when near, others drop to a hare only the most desirable manner of pointing is with the head and tail up, but all cease to move when very near

There is no doubt any Dog possessing a good nose may be taught to point ; instances occur of the Terrier and Spaniel, yet none seem so appropriate to the purpose as the Spanish Dog, whose instinct is entirely directed to that, and whose education is easy.

The most judicious cross appears to have been with the Fox Hound, as by this has been acquired speed and courage, power and perseverance; and its disadvantage, difficulty of training them to be staunch. I believe the celebrated Colonel Thornton first made this cross, and from his producing excellent Dogs, has been very generally followed.

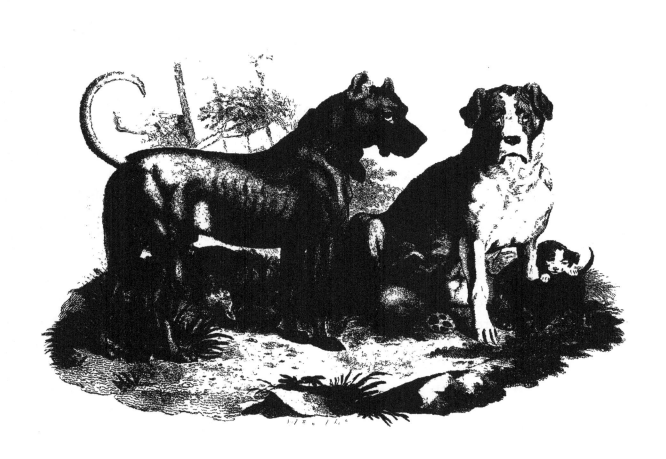

CANIS MASTIVUS.

THE MASTIFF.

Canis Villaticus, seu Catinarius, Mastive or Bandedog —CAIUS.
Le Dogue de forte race —BUFF.
Canis Mastivus.—RAII
Canis Molossus —LINN.
Canis Molossus Bellicosus Anglicus, Mastiff —CHARLTON.
English Dogue —RIDINGER

OF a very powerful make, twenty-eight or thirty inches high, broad chest, head large, lips pendulous and thick, ears small and hanging down, tail thin, coat short and smooth, colour all tanned or brindled with a black muzzle, a dark spot over each eye, or these colours varied with white. I have examined several of them, and found them uniformly a little underhung, the lower jaw beyond the upper. His race is disseminated over all the continent, one or two I have seen brought to England were very large and strong, but not so tall as those I remember here; their heads were shorter, colour black and tan; in other respects they were exactly like ours, and are often figured in the prints of Ridinger with the Dane, and appear to have been used for similar purposes.

What the Lion is to the Cat the Mastiff is to the Dog, the noblest of the family; he stands alone, and all others sink before him. His courage does not exceed his temper and generosity, and in attachment he equals the kindest of his race. His docility is perfect, the teazing of the smaller kinds will hardly provoke him to resent, and I have seen him hold down with his paw the Terrier or Cur that has bit him, without offering further injury. In a family he will permit the children to play with him, and suffer all their little pranks without offence. The blind ferocity of the Bull Dog will often wound the hand of the master who assists him to combat, but the Mastiff distinguishes perfectly, enters the field with temper, and engages in the attack as if confident of success: if he overpowers, or is beaten, his master may take him immediately in his arms and fear nothing. This ancient and faithful domestic, the pride of our island, uniting the useful, the brave, and the docile, though sought by foreign nations and perpetuated on the continent, is nearly extinct where he probably was an aborigine, or is bastardised by numberless crosses, every one of which degenerate from the invaluable character of the parent, who was deemed worthy to enter the Roman amphitheatre, and, in the presence of the masters of the world, encounter the pard, and assail even the lord of the savage tribes, whose courage was sublimed by torrid suns, and found none gallant enough to oppose him on the deserts of Zaara or the plains of Numidia.

The Romans, according to Camden, appointed an officer to reside in Britain, with the title of Procurator Cynegii, whose sole business was to breed and transmit from hence such Dogs as were deemed equal to the combat of the amphitheatre; his station was at Winchester. In Scotland they must have been in great perfection Symmachus, speaking of seven brought from that country, says, " they were observed to be so fierce at the games, that they universally imagined them to have been brought over in cages of iron." Provoking the Mastiff to this degree of fury would naturally be a theatrical trick of the procurers to strike the spectators. The fierce northern nations, who settled in Gaul, in their barbarous mode of warfare, embattled them for the fight; thus the Colophoni and Castabalenses formed the front line of their armies with dogs, and after the defeat of the Cimbri by Marius, the dogs defended the baggage for some time against the victorious Romans. Shakspeare might allude to this when he says, " Cry havock, and let slip the dogs of war."

Our rude and illiterate, but intrepid and generous ancestors, do not appear to have used the Mastiff in war; nor is it likely that they, who, in all ages, have reared their brave breasts, and fought foot to foot in the battle, would chuse such an ally, however courageous. The chieftain placed a warder in the watch tower to notice by blowing his horn the approach of a visitor, or any martial excursion; the property of the chief was safe, being in the midst of his vassals, and the mere serfs would hardly maintain so expensive a guard for their flocks. For what then was this dog so attentively bred in this island as to be an object of admiration on the continent; sought for the theatrical hunt by the Romans, and for war by the cunning and ferocious Gaul? Ancient Albion and mountainous Caledonia were covered with thick and extensive forests, in which wandered at will the wolf, the bear, the boar, and mountain bull, the probable ancestor of our domestic cattle; the inhabitants, subsisting on the milk of their flocks, and the flesh of wild or domestic animals, in the intervals of their numerous wars would have little employment but the hunt; this would be their continued refuge from the listlessness of inactivity and the prelude to every entertainment. I have already stated that the ancient hunt was very different to our present refined, and I may say comparatively effeminate, chase of the smaller animals; when the Game started it was brought to bay and assailed by the hunter himself, whose life was ever in danger; what could be nobler sport to the heroic chieftain than the attack of the wild bull?

MASTIFF.

Through the huge oaks of Evandale,
   Whose limbs a thousand years have worn,
What sullen roar comes down the gale,
   And drowns the hunter's pealing horn?

Mightiest of all the beasts of chase,
   That roam in woody Caledon,
Crashing the forest in his race,
   The mountain bull comes thundering on.

Fierce on the hunter's quiver'd band
   He rolls his eyes of swarthy glow,
Spurns with black hoof and horn the sand,
   And tosses high his mane of snow

Aim'd well, the chieftain's lance has flown,
   Struggling in blood the savage lies,
His roar is sunk in hollow groan—
   Sound, merry huntsmen, sound the *pryse*.

Our historians mention the danger of these hunts; Robert Bruce was preserved from the rage of a wild bull by a courtier, who from thence acquired for himself and lineage the name of Turn-Bull; Fitzstephen mentions them as inhabiting the great forest that lay adjacent to London in his day; and Sibbald, as covering the mountains of Scotland, where they are still preserved by the Duke of Montrose. If the chieftain's lance was unfortunate, the wild bull, like the bos and bison, would precipitate himself against the hunter and his horse; this would be the moment of associating the Mastiff in the chase, to divert the fury of the bull, and preserve the hunter, as he is not to be bayed; thence would he be the companion of every hunt, protected, and caressed; thence the cultivation of his courage, and his fearlessly rushing to the combat in the Roman amphitheatre. Manwood,

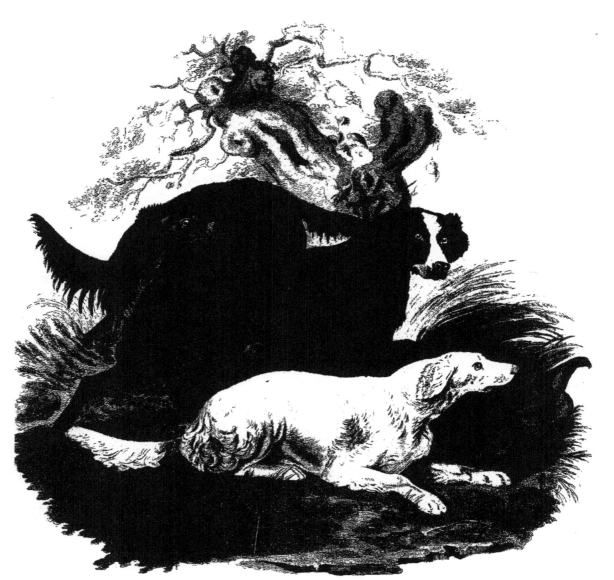